A gap in therapy for ADHD has been beautifully addressed by this program for managing executive functioning deficits in the college student population. The authors, all experts in adult ADHD, have distilled their years of clinical research and expertise into a finely-honed program, a necessary resource for anyone working with this ADHD population.

Russell A. Barkley, Ph.D. *Clinical Neuropsychologist, Retired. Author,*
Taking Charge of ADHD *and* Taking Charge of Adult ADHD

A great resource! It takes foundational skills that have been validated in adults and in high school students and applies them to the unique needs of college students. Modules including "adulting," substance use, balancing independence with looping in parents, and next steps in the workplace make this highly relevant. I would highly recommend this program to any clinician working with college students coping with full-fledged ADHD or with related symptoms.

Steven A. Safren, Ph.D. *Professor of Psychology, University of Miami. Author,* Mastering Your Adult ADHD:
A Cognitive-Behavioral Treatment Program

Thriving in College with ADHD is the right program at the right time for the field. The therapist guide offers a modular structure grounded in rigorous science with flexibility to meet individual client needs. The accompanying student workbook for clients is inviting and user-friendly. The package helps clinicians transform science into action. Exactly what university counseling centers need right now.

Julie S. Owens, Ph.D. *Professor of Psychology and Co-Director of the Center for Intervention Research in Schools, Ohio University*

W01113709

THRIVING IN COLLEGE WITH ADHD

Thriving in College with ADHD uses cognitive-behavioral and psychoeducational techniques to address ADHD and related impairments in a way that is tailored to the needs of college students.

This manual distills the expertise of four psychologists with extensive experience helping students with ADHD. The treatment is designed to be effective, flexible, and feasible. Modules address organization, time management, planning, academic skills, adaptive thinking, healthy lifestyles, relationships, and other life skills. They can be used with individuals or groups and as an abbreviated or comprehensive treatment, tailored to client needs. The accompanying student workbook will increase the treatment's impact and keep college students engaged in learning new skills.

Any mental health professional working with college students with ADHD can benefit their clients by adding this approach to their toolbox.

Will Canu, Ph.D., is a Professor of Psychology at Appalachian State University. His research focuses mainly on ADHD in adulthood, including adjustment, assessment, and interventions.

Laura E. Knouse, Ph.D. is a Professor of Psychology at the University of Richmond. She is an expert in CBT for adult ADHD and study skills for college students with ADHD.

Kate Flory, Ph.D. is a Professor of Psychology at the University of South Carolina. She studies social, emotional, health, academic, and other outcomes among children, adolescents, and young adults with ADHD.

Cynthia M. Hartung, Ph.D. is a Professor of Psychology at the University of Wyoming. She studies the assessment and treatment of ADHD in adolescents and emerging adults and sex/gender differences in psychopathology.

Thriving in College with ADHD

A Cognitive-Behavioral Skills Manual for Therapists

Will Canu, Laura E. Knouse, Kate Flory, and Cynthia M. Hartung

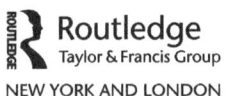

Routledge
Taylor & Francis Group

NEW YORK AND LONDON

Cover image: © Getty Images

First published 2024
by Routledge
605 Third Avenue, New York, NY 10158

and by Routledge
4 Park Square, Milton Park, Abingdon, Oxon, OX14 4RN

Routledge is an imprint of the Taylor & Francis Group, an informa business

ISBN: 978-0-367-71161-0 (hbk)
ISBN: 978-0-367-71160-3 (pbk)
ISBN: 978-1-003-14959-0 (ebk)

DOI: 10.4324/9781003149590

Typeset in Baskerville
by MPS Limited, Dehradun

Contents

Acknowledgments   *xi*

Introduction for Therapists   1

Educating Clients *(~2 sessions)* – Corresponds to the
Introduction of the *Thriving in College* Student Workbook   10

1   ADHD, EF Deficits, and Other Issues that Impact
    Concentration   11

2   Psychosocial and Medication Treatments for ADHD   21

Skill 1: Organization, Time Management, and Planning
Skills *(~4 sessions)* – Corresponds to Skillset 1 in the *Thriving
in College* Student Workbook   31

1   Choosing a Calendar and Task List System –
    Corresponds to Modules 1.0 and 1.1 in the
    Thriving in College Student Workbook   34

2   Beginning and Continuing to Use a Calendar and Task
    List System – Corresponds to Module 1.2 in the *Thriving
    in College* Student Workbook   43

3 Task Prioritization and Sustaining Behavior through Rewards and Accountability – Corresponds to Modules 1.3 and 1.4 in the *Thriving in College* Student Workbook   52

4 Managing Procrastination – Corresponds to Module 1.5 in the *Thriving in College* Student Workbook   60

Skill 2: Becoming a Professional Learner *(1-2 sessions)* – Corresponds to Skillset 2 of the *Thriving in College* Student Workbook   67

1 Implement New Academic Skills – Corresponds to Modules 2.0–2.6 in the *Thriving in College* Student Workbook   70

2 Follow-up and Academic Support and Accommodations – Corresponds to Module 2.6 in the *Thriving in College* Student Workbook   88

Skill 3: Thinking and Responding Differently *(~4 sessions)* – Corresponds to Skillset 3 of the *Thriving in College* Student Workbook   96

1 Being Mindful – Corresponds to Module 3.1 in the *Thriving in College* Student Workbook   102

2 Noticing Your Patterns – Corresponds to Module 3.2 in the *Thriving in College* Student Workbook   114

3 Practicing New Responses – Corresponds to Module 3.3 in the *Thriving in College* Student Workbook   123

4 Managing Strong Emotions and Impulsive Behavior – Corresponds to Module 3.4 in the *Thriving in College* Student Workbook   133

Skill 4: Taking Good Care of Yourself *(~3 sessions)* –
Corresponds to Skillset 4 of the *Thriving in College*
Student Workbook   142

1   How is ADHD Related to Sleep, Nutrition, Physical
     Activity, Substance Use, Technology Use, and Driving? –
     Corresponds to Module 4.0 in the *Thriving in College*
     Student Workbook   144

2   Identifying Health-related Behaviors for Goal Setting –
     Corresponds to Modules 4.1–4.6 in the *Thriving in College*
     Student Workbook   153

3   Strategies for Improving Sleep, Eating Healthier,
     Increasing Physical Activity, Managing Substance and
     Technology Use, and Driving Safely – Corresponds to
     Modules 4.1–4.6 in the *Thriving in College* Student
     Workbook   159

Skill 5: Being Successful in Relationships *(~3 sessions)* –
Corresponds to Skillset 5 of the *Thriving in College* Student
Workbook   168

1   Learning About Relationships, Relationship Skills, and
     ADHD – Corresponds to Module 5.0 of the *Thriving in
     College* Student Workbook   175

2   Changing Behaviors to be Satisfied in My Personal
     Relationships – Corresponds to Module 5.1 of the
     Thriving in College Student Workbook   183

3   (Re)negotiating a Positive Relationship with Parents –
     Corresponds to Module 5.2 of the *Thriving in College*
     Student Workbook   195

Skill 6: Managing Tasks of Daily Living or "Adulting" *(~3 sessions)* – Corresponds to Skillset 6 of the *Thriving in College* Student Workbook   208

1   How ADHD is Related to Impairment in Daily Life Activities and Identifying Areas for Improvement – Corresponds to Module 6.0 of the *Thriving in College* Student Workbook   210

2   Strategies for Effectively Managing Important Life Activities – Corresponds to Module 6.1–6.3 of the *Thriving in College* Student Workbook   216

3   Succeeding at Work and Crafting a Career – Corresponds to Module 6.4 of the *Thriving in College* Student Workbook   221

   Appendix A: Handouts for Clients   *230*
   Appendix B: Assessment Scales   *259*
   Index   *288*

Acknowledgments

We express our sincere gratitude to the graduate students in our labs and on our practicum teams who helped to lead the therapy groups on which this approach is based. We also wish to thank our clients whose hard work and insights have informed this work and made it better. We also thank Alex Fossum for her assistance with graphic design and manuscript formatting.

Thank you to Rebekah for all of your support and encouragement, and thank you to Owen and Sophia, for being my Sun and Moon. You inspire me, and I love you all more than words can say. -WC

Many thanks to my undergraduate research students who gave helpful feedback on my draft material during the completion of this work and to the University of Richmond for their support via a School of Arts and Sciences Faculty Summer Research Fellowship and a Faculty Fellowship from the Office of the Provost. -LEK

Special thanks to the University of South Carolina College of Arts and Sciences for their support via a Book Manuscript Finalization Award. All my love to my family, Neil, Carter, and Austin, who support me fully in everything that I do. -KF

I am grateful to my graduate students, Christopher, Patrick, Anne, Judah, John, and Tamara, who contributed their ingenious ideas to this program over the years. Working with you all is the best part of my job. Love and thanks to Billie and Ben, who have both appreciated and tolerated my planning skills especially during their school years when they allowed me to try out many of these techniques with them and gave me honest feedback. -CMH

Introduction for Therapists

As should be obvious from its title, this treatment manual is, primarily, an attempt to provide clinicians and clinical researchers our detailed and empirically informed perspective on intervention with college students with attention-deficit/hyperactivity disorder (ADHD). Over the course of the past few decades, it has become accepted that ADHD occurs not only in children and adolescents but also in adults. The field has responded accordingly, and several clinical researchers have done groundbreaking work (e.g., Steve Safren, Ph.D., Susan Sprich, Ph.D., Mary Solanto, Ph.D., Russell Barkley, Ph.D., Russell Ramsay, M.D., Margaret Weiss, M.D., Arthur Anastopoulos, Ph.D., Andrea Chronis-Tuscano, Ph.D., Joshua Langberg, Ph.D.) to both understand how ADHD is manifested in adulthood and how we can address its related impairments in psychotherapy. In general, approaches that emphasize (a) psychoeducation regarding ADHD and pharmacological treatment, (b) behavioral training of adaptive skills, and (c) cognitive techniques that help mitigate emotional and inhibitory dysfunctions have been shown to help affected adults to be better adjusted in school, work, and other domains of life (Knouse, 2015; Kooij et al., 2010; Safren et al., 2010; Solanto et al., 2010).

Given this situation, you may ask why it is that another treatment manual is needed. The most parsimonious answer is this: There is a dearth of published treatment protocols for college students with ADHD, and this represents a subpopulation that merits special attention. Behavioral parent training, summer and after-school treatment programs, and other classroom-based and pharmacological interventions have been studied and validated for children, and cognitive-behavioral and medical approaches have garnered substantial empirical support for use in mature adults (i.e., mid-thirties and up), as well. The net result is a set of published and thereby readily implementable psychosocial treatment procedures for younger and older individuals with the disorder, but a relative void for emerging adult clients (i.e., those who are 18 to 25 years old). Further, while there is evidence to suggest that those individuals with ADHD who do matriculate to college may, overall, have relatively less-severe symptoms than their same-aged peers who choose not to pursue (or are not admitted to)

DOI: 10.4324/9781003149590-1

higher education, many in the former group will leave the structure and comfort of their family home, move across their state or even the country, and attempt to establish themselves in relative independence in pursuing higher education. They leave behind the supervision of parents, the assistance of teachers and possibly psychotherapists, and the routines and organization that they developed or were imposed by others that helped them to at least academically succeed through high school. This all occurs at a developmental juncture that poses risks even for those who are not already burdened by ADHD. It is therefore not surprising that a much higher percentage of college students with ADHD —well over 50% by some accounts— fail to complete a degree as compared to their non-diagnosed counterparts (Murphy et al., 2002). Yet it is painfully clear, given economic and other data that is readily available, that completion of a college degree in today's world is strongly associated with positive outcomes, such as job security, health, and overall well-being.

As such and given our collective experience in both treating and researching the difficulties that are faced by this select group, we believe that there is a need for this manual. Furthermore, there is a need for the wide dissemination of effective treatment procedures specifically for college students with ADHD, to help them to succeed in their educational goals, to be better adapted in social and eventual work settings, and also to experience less personal distress related to the combination of their inherent behavioral challenges and the demands of higher education and independent living. Successful pursuit of this goal via the use of this manual requires specialized, graduate-level training in professional psychology or counseling, as is achieved with degrees such as the Ph.D., Psy.D., MD, DSW, MSW, and counseling and clinical psychology MAs. Whether you are a professional therapist at a university counseling center, a staff member of a university-based psychology clinic, a physician or nursing professional at student health services, a counselor working with disability or learning assistance services, or an independent practitioner working with college or college-bound students, we believe that the techniques noted herein will help you to provide effective services for your clients.

Assessment and Treatment Planning

As clinical psychologists, we have been trained to let data guide our practice, both in terms of the interventions we choose to employ and the identification of clients' individual goals. Depending on the setting that you practice in, formal assessment may be emphasized or de-emphasized. There are realities regarding personnel resources and factors that might preclude formal diagnostic assessment of some or even all clients, and treatment planning may occur "on the fly." Regardless of the depth or frequency of initial assessments in your setting, we strongly recommend using at least brief measures of symptoms and impairment when treating college students with ADHD.

ADHD symptom reports abound, and vary from pay-per-use, self-scoring measures (e.g., Conner's Adult ADHD Rating Scales; Conners, Erhardt, & Sparrow, 1999) to questionnaires that are available for purchase but can be reproduced for professional use thereafter (e.g., Barkley Adult ADHD Rating Scale-IV; Barkley, 2014) to public domain scales (Adult ADHD Self-Report Scale v. 1.1, ASRS, Kessler et al., 2005). Establishing a baseline for the severity of each client's ADHD symptoms and follow-up with these brief assessments throughout and at the end of treatment will help you and your clients to gauge improvement regarding their underlying deficits. Further, some research (e.g., Penberthy et al., 2012) substantiates the general clinical wisdom regarding community-based diagnoses of ADHD: while it is likely that most of such decisions regarding the presence of ADHD are accurate, there certainly is a proportion that is not. It is not our purpose to outline or debate the reasons for such inaccuracy, but instead to reinforce the use of symptom reports to help corroborate the presence of ADHD when a client presents with a reported prior diagnosis, and particularly when this is presented without supporting documentation.

It is important for the therapist to note that leaders in the field (e.g., Biederman et al., 2006; Gathje, Lewandowski, & Gordon, 2008) and ADHD treatment outcome studies in general have been placing increasing emphasis on the assessment of functional adaptation, relative to improvement, in core ADHD symptomatology. As with many trends in adult ADHD research, this stems from reflection regarding outcomes after psychosocial intervention with affected children. For instance, the initial results of the Multimodal Treatment for ADHD (MTA) study, the largest randomized controlled trial of active ADHD interventions conducted to date, suggested that highly organized and well-titrated stimulant medication treatment outperformed behavior therapy, combined therapy (i.e., behavior therapy + stimulant medication), and community-care medication management (MTA Cooperative Group, 1999). However, these conclusions were based on short-term follow-up and examination of symptom reports. Subsequently, more discerning analyses that examined the functional adaptation of these children across life domains and time have yielded a different picture. For instance, Langberg and colleagues (2010) document how, in adaptive behavior of homework completion, MTA treatments including behavior therapy (i.e., behavior therapy and combined) produce great and more durable improvement, as compared to medication alone. As this illustrates, symptom improvement alone should not be the goal of intervention—there should be an equal focus on mitigated functional impairment. As such, we strongly urge therapists employing our treatment modules to include brief measures of functional adaptation at baseline and intervals throughout intervention—for example, the Tracker scale located in the Appendix. Other adaptive functioning measures that are specific to ADHD include the Weiss Functional Impairment Rating Scale (Weiss, 2000) and the Barkley Functional Impairment Rating Scale (Barkley, 2011).

A Cognitive-Behavioral Model of ADHD

The cognitive-behavioral model developed by Safren and colleagues (2004) describes how living with ADHD symptoms both interferes with behavioral self-regulation strategies and generates perceived failure experiences that contribute to dysfunctional thoughts and beliefs. ADHD is not caused by behaviors and thoughts, but the degree to which people can cope effectively with their symptoms and reach their goals in the context of their ADHD depends upon learning and practicing effective behavioral and cognitive self-regulation strategies. Like the work of Safren et al. (2004), our treatment targets both behavioral and cognitive processes. Figure 1 illustrates a simplified cognitive-behavioral model of ADHD and this treatment.

In this treatment, college students with ADHD learn to implement self-regulation skills such as organization, time management, and planning skills, into their daily lives and practice them until they can become less effortful. Later, they are also coached to become more aware of the thinking patterns that can get in the way of using skills and staying motivated and then engage in practicing new ways of thinking and responding in challenging situations and in the presence of challenging emotions. As such, our treatment addresses both behavioral and cognitive contributors to functional impairments in college students with ADHD.

As with any form of cognitive-behavioral therapy, it is important to ensure that the client clearly understands the rationale for treatment and how it can

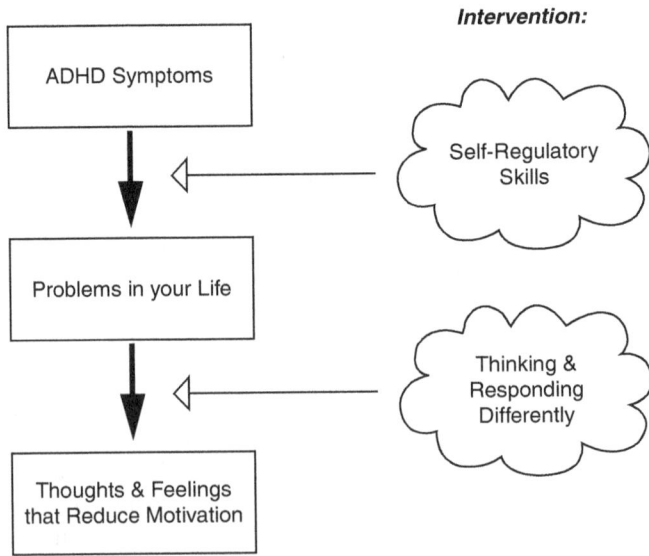

Figure 1 Simplified model of CBT for adult ADHD.

help them meet their goals. During the assessment process or during the first session, clinicians should engage each client in an interactive discussion about the cognitive-behavioral model of ADHD and how the skills learned in CBT can help them improve their lives. Clients should also be prepared with information on what to expect from their therapist, what will be expected of them, and how to make the most of treatment. Above all, clinicians should foster a *growth mindset* about the client's ability to learn and implement new self-regulation skills and express confidence in the potential for positive change.

While experienced CBT practitioners will likely have their own strategies and language for conveying this information, clinicians should emphasize the following points supported by Figure 1.

1 Living with ADHD often causes problems in a person's life and living with those problems over time can lead to ways of thinking and feeling that negatively impact motivation to overcome ADHD.
2 CBT will involve **learning new self-regulation skills** to help reduce the extent to which ADHD symptoms cause problems.
3 CBT will also involve **learning to recognize how your thoughts and feelings affect your motivation** and **learning how to respond differently.**
4 Like any new skill, CBT skills will require consistent practice to master. Practice in the "real world" is essential, so there will be homework.
5 The client may need to try out different strategies and tweak them to fit them into their lifestyle. There may be some trial and error.
6 You will help the client set specific goals for reducing the negative impact of ADHD symptoms and monitor progress toward those goals.
7 Progress may be slow at times and there will be setbacks, but you are prepared to work with the client to persevere.

How to Implement This Modular Treatment

We have intentionally formatted this intervention in modules to facilitate flexible and responsive implementation that can be tailored to the individual needs of college student clients. That being said, based on our extensive clinical and research experience, **we strongly urge practitioners to employ Modules One (Psychoeducation) and Two (Organization, time management, and planning skills) as a standard, "starter" treatment package, for the following reasons**.

First, it is always surprising to us how many college students with prior ADHD diagnoses have little background knowledge of their condition, or perhaps worse, inaccurate knowledge. This may come about for reasonable developmental reasons, as many are diagnosed early in childhood and may either not remember what they were told then or were left out of therapist-parent interpretive sessions at the end of assessment. Such students may only know (a) that they have been diagnosed with ADHD and (b) that they are supposed to take their medication to address the symptoms. While this might be enough for functional adaptation in best-case scenarios (i.e., medication addresses symptoms well and adherence is never an issue), this commonly represents a serious hurdle to success in treatment and in life and in developing an accurate and positive self-regard. "I never knew that" and "I wish someone had told me this years ago" are common refrains from clients, and the insights that they gain into the underlying causes of their cognitive and behavioral symptoms, their likely course, and the common functional problems that all with people with ADHD face often facilitate motivation in the treatment and a decrease in the negative self-talk that exacerbates the impact of core symptoms.

Second, the greatest challenge that all college students face is the multi-faceted endeavor of mastering independent living and adjustment in an intellectually and organizationally challenging milieu. Gone are the highly structured days of high school, where teachers and administrators helped to keep one on task and in the right location and, often, provided special in-class learning accommodations. For many, this transition also involves shedding the assistance and organization provided by concerned parents or other guardians. No one is there to help the budding adult to start and focus on homework after class. No one is there to ensure that steps are taken early enough to complete term projects. No one is there to meter out dollars on a strict need-to-have basis. For any student, assuming all the responsibility that such independence entails can be difficult, if not overwhelming. However, for those affected by ADHD, all of this is so much harder (Fleming & McMahon, 2012). Most of the college students that we see in our clinics are beset with problems related to poor organization and judgment when it comes to task planning and completion and day-to-day self-care, and this quite often results in a major adaptive problem: low grades that result in probation or expulsion. Given that successful completion of coursework is, by definition, the main purpose of attending college, Module Two is for many a critical lifeline to needed skill development.

Aside from these modules that we regard as centrally important, the therapist is encouraged to use the client's developmental stage as well as data from clinical interviews and, we hope, functional impairment measures to guide the choice and timing of additional modules.

A word of caution: collective clinical experience suggests that treatment duration is an important consideration, and we have found that this is especially true for college students. For various reasons including semester schedules, the strong pull of social and extracurricular activities, the way that academic demands surge and ebb, and the need of many students to work jobs to support their education, client attendance and treatment adherence in interventions that last more than six-to-eight weeks can be problematic. The core treatment that we recommend (Modules One and Two) will typically last 4 to 7 sessions, which we have found to be quite feasible and tolerable for college students. As such, adding one more module to a dose of psychosocial intervention seems like a reasonable idea, and the therapist can customize their client's treatment thusly based on their most critical, identified need.

Of course, you may encounter clients who could benefit from all the modules that we detail in this manual. You may be practicing in a setting (e.g., university counseling center) where you have many clients with diverse needs, and consequently wonder how you can successfully provide tailored intervention for so many students. In both cases, our advice is consistent: focus first on providing the psychoeducation and organization, time management, and planning (OTMP) pieces and then figure out how other, needed aspects can be delivered as add-ons that require only short-term attendance. For instance, in a counseling center you might offer a psychoeducation and OTMP group, then encourage individual therapists to follow up with their clients as indicated over time with content from other modules. Alternatively, after the first group, you might in the next term offer a cognitive strategies (Module Six) group and a social relationships group (Module Seven), both of which are short term and allows freedom of choice and at a minimal cost of therapist time.

A final note: one thing that we strongly suggest and encourage, no matter what setting you are in, that you regard implementing this protocol as an iterative process and, as such, that you collect and use data regarding the outcomes of your clients. While we obviously view it as positive for guiding the field, we do not mean to imply that you need to publish your achieved results. What we wish is that you use this intervention in an empirically informed way. Your emphasis with current clients may change for the better, as may your approach with future clients. Try it. We think you will like it, and that your clients will appreciate that you care to measure their progress and adapt as needed. We have included a brief measure, called the *Progress Tracker*, in Appendix B, that measures impairment for college students with ADHD. We recommend that you track your client's progress and adaptation in college using this measure, employing it at the beginning of every session. Of course, you may choose to use other treatment outcome measures, as well, depending on your clients' individual issues and needs.

Student Workbook

To guide the treatment and make it more accessible to both clients and therapists, we have created an accompanying student workbook: *Thriving in College with ADHD: Student Workbook*. Use of the workbook in administering this treatment is optional; however, it can provide clients with additional opportunities for psychoeducation and skills practice and serve as a complement to in-session work and homework assignments set by the therapist.

To facilitate the integration of the workbook into treatment, we reference corresponding workbook skillsets and modules throughout this therapist guide. Note that the workbook often breaks skill sections down into smaller "chunks," and so a single session in this therapist guide may correspond to multiple modules in the workbook.

References

Barkley, R.A. (2011). *Barkley functional impairment rating scale (BFIS for adults)*. Guilford Press.

Barkley, R.A. (2014). *Barkley adult ADHD rating scale-IV (BAARS-IV)*. Guilford Press.

Biederman, J., Faraone, S. V., Spencer, T. J., Mick, E., Monuteaux, M. C., & Aleardi, M. (2006). Functional impairments in adults with self-reports of diagnosed ADHD: A controlled study of 1001 adults in the community. *The Journal of Clinical Psychiatry, 67*(4), 524–540. 10.4088/jcp.v67n0403

Conners, C.K., Erhardt, D., & Sparrow, E.P. (1999). *Conners' adult ADHD rating scales: Technical manual*. New York: Multi-Health Systems.

Fleming, A.P., & McMahon, R.J. (2012). Developmental context and treatment principles for ADHD among college students. *Clinical Child and Family Psychology Review, 15*(4), 303–329. 10.1007/s10567-012-0121-z

Gathje, R. A., Lewandowski, L. J., & Gordon, M. (2008). The role of impairment in the diagnosis of ADHD. *Journal of Attention Disorders, 11*(5), 529–537. 10.1177/1087054 707314028

Kessler, R.C., Adler, L., Ames, M., Demler, O., Faraone, S., Hiripi, E., Howes, M.J., Jin, R., Secnik, K., Spencer, T., Ustun, T.B., & Walters, E.E. (2005). The World Health Organization Adult ADHD Self-Report Scale (ASRS): A short screening scale for use in the general population. *Psychological Medicine, 35*(2), 245–256. 10.1017/ s0033291704002892

Knouse, L.E. (2015). Cognitive-Behavioral Therapy for ADHD in College: Recommendations "Hot Off the Press". *The ADHD Report, 23*(5), 8–15. 10.1521/adhd.2015. 23.5.8

Kooij, S.J., Bejerot, S., Blackwell, A., et al. (2010). European consensus statement on diagnosis and treatment of adult ADHD: The European Network Adult ADHD. *BMC Psychiatry, 10*, 67. 10.1186/1471-244X-10-67

Langberg, J. M., Arnold, L. E., Flowers, A. M., Epstein, J. N., Altaye, M., Hinshaw, S. P., Swanson, J. M., Kotkin, R., Simpson, S., Molina, B. S., Jensen, P. S., Abikoff, H., Pelham, W. E., Jr, Vitiello, B., Wells, K. C., & Hechtman, L. (2010). Parent-reported homework problems in the MTA study: evidence for sustained improvement with behavioral treatment. *Journal of Clinical Child and Adolescent Psychology, 39*(2), 220–233. 10.1 080/15374410903532700

MTA Cooperative Group. (1999). A 14-month randomized clinical trial of treatment strategies for attention-deficit/hyperactivity disorder. Multimodal Treatment Study of Children with ADHD. *Archives of General Psychiatry, 56*(12), 1073–1086. 10.1001/ archpsyc.5612.1073 PMID: 10591283.

Murphy, K.R., Barkley, R.A., & Bush, T. (2002). Young adults with attention deficit hyperactivity disorder: Differences in comorbidity, educational, and clinical history. *The Journal of Nervous and Mental Disease, 190*(3), 147–157. 10.1097/00005053-200203000-00003

Penberthy, J.K., Breton, M.D., Runyon, C.F., & Kovatchev, B.P. (2012). Retrospective analysis of ADHD diagnoses in an outpatient pediatric clinic. *Journal of Ethics in Mental Health*, *7*(1), 1–5. Retrieved from https://jemh.ca/issues/v7/JEMHVol72012.html

Safren, S.A., Sprich, S., Chulvick, S., & Otto, M.W. (2004). Psychosocial treatments for adults with attention-deficit/hyperactivity disorder. *The Psychiatric Clinics of North America*, *27*(2), 349–360. 10.1016/S0193-953X(03)00089-3

Safren, S.A., Sprich, S., Mimiaga, M.J., Surman, C., Knouse, L., Groves, M., & Otto, M.W. (2010). Cognitive behavioral therapy vs relaxation with educational support for medication-treated adults with ADHD and persistent symptoms: A randomized controlled trial. *Journal of the American Medical Association*, *304*(8), 875–880. 10.1001/jama.2010.1192

Solanto, M.V., Marks, D.J., Wasserstein, J., Mitchell, K., Abikoff, H., Alvir, J.M., & Kofman, M.D. (2010). Efficacy of meta-cognitive therapy for adult ADHD. *The American Journal of Psychiatry*, *167*(8), 958–968. 10.1176/appi.ajp.2009.09081123

Weiss, M.D. (2000). *Weiss Functional Impairment Rating Scale (WFIRS) Self-Report*. Vancouver, Canada: University of British Columbia. Retrieved from naceonline.com/AdultADHDtoolkit/assessmenttools/wfirs.pdf

Educating Clients

(~2 sessions)

Corresponds to the Introduction of the *Thriving in College* Student Workbook

Background for the Therapist

In these sessions, you will be educating your client(s) about the following topics:

- ADHD and executive functioning (EF) deficits
- Other things that look like ADHD
- Psychotherapy including interventions and training
- Medication treatment of ADHD

Much of the content that you will find in these sessions mirrors what you have learned by reading the introductory material for therapists earlier in this manual. As outlined herein, the topics that are included can be discussed with students in a group, individual or combined individual-and-group therapy format. We recommend that these psychoeducation topics be introduced and discussed during two therapy sessions, as organized below, but, depending on the duration of sessions, three meetings might be necessary.

You should note that the content provided below is mainly to facilitate didactic presentation to your client(s). In other words, unlike in the "skills" sections of this manual, there is not a lot of instruction or "technique" for you to directly use. Use the included material as a basis for presentation to or discussion with your client(s) regarding the nature and treatment of ADHD. PowerPoint or similar visual aids and organization are recommended.

Student Workbook

If you are using the *Thriving in College* student workbook, you will find that Part 1 of the Introduction on *Understanding ADHD* partially covers the material in Sessions 1 and 2 of this section but in less comprehensive detail. Part 2 of the introduction guides students through exercises from motivational interviewing to help set the stage for the skills-based work to come. You may wish to assign workbook Part 2: Get Motivated as part of your client's homework following the first or section session.

DOI: 10.4324/9781003149590-2

Session 1: ADHD, EF Deficits, and Other Issues that Impact Concentration

Session Outline

1 Check-in with client(s)
2 Set agenda
3 What is attention-deficit/hyperactivity disorder?
4 What are executive functioning problems?
5 What else could be causing you to have difficulty concentrating?
6 How is ADHD assessed?
7 General discussion
8 Discuss homework
9 Schedule next session

Session Organization

Administration Format

Session 1 can be administered in a group or individual format. A group session is optimal because students often benefit from sharing their struggles with ADHD and related impairment, and also because of added efficiency in educating several clients at once. In addition to providing the opportunity for support, encouragement, and modeling, research suggests that clients who interact with others who have ADHD have reduced stigma toward ADHD (Chew, Jensen & Rosen, 2009). Nonetheless, an individual session is acceptable if a group session is not indicated or practical.

Materials and Preparation Needed

The therapist should have the following materials available for this session.

- A whiteboard, flipchart, or a projected digital document to capture group ideas and/or present material
- A list of "take home messages" regarding the session's content as well as instructions/goals for at-home work prior to the next session

DOI: 10.4324/9781003149590-3

Qualified therapists who do not feel fully conversant in the etiology and characteristics of ADHD are instructed to study background material before commencing this first session of the psychoeducation module (e.g., *Attention-Deficit Hyperactivity Disorder: A Handbook for Diagnosis & Treatment* [4th edition], Barkley, 2015; *ADHD in Adults: What the Science Says*, Barkley, Murphy, & Fischer, 2008). Therapists may similarly wish to prepare and provide reference lists of more "popular" literature on ADHD (e.g., *Driven to Distraction (Revised): Recognizing and Coping with Attention Deficit Disorder*, Hallowell & Ratey, 2011) and handouts with empirically supported information for clients (e.g., those available through the National Institute of Mental Health, at https://www.nimh.nih.gov/health/publications/adhd-what-you-need-to-know). Finally, you will want to instruct clients ahead of the session to bring a notebook or device on which they can take notes.

Session Content

Check in with Client(s)

Check-in time can be used to solicit brief discussion, or simply to see how things are going and build rapport. In the event that this session is the first meeting with clients, check-in might focus more on feelings and expectations about therapy. In any event, aim for this to be brief (< 5 minutes), encouraging for any additional discussion of this sort to be postponed until after the session content is completed. See therapist-client check-in dialog example in Skill 1: Session 1 as a model for this interaction, if needed. We also recommend having your client complete the *Progress Tracker* (see Appendix B), and briefly touching base on any declines or improvements in school functioning.

Set Agenda

Introduce the agenda for this session to the client (see above). It may be helpful to have a visual aid to refer to, such as a flip chart or projected PowerPoint slide or printed handout. At this time, it might also be helpful to remind clients to write notes regarding important points in a therapy notebook. Setting the agenda should be speedily completed (< 2 minutes). See therapist-client agenda-setting dialog example in Skill 1: Session 1 as a model, if needed.

What Is Attention-Deficit/Hyperactivity Disorder (ADHD)?

If the clients you are treating have been diagnosed with ADHD (or have been treated for this previously) or are deemed to be at risk for this disorder, psychoeducation regarding its nature is critical. It is important to realize that such students, even those with longstanding and well-established ADHD diagnoses, will have varying levels of understanding regarding the underlying nature of ADHD.

Some may have been told in early childhood by their parents that they have ADHD and may only know that taking medication helps them do better in school. Others may have wondered for quite some time about whether ADHD might be getting in their way in school or other areas of life and may just now be coming to learn more about it. Even students who think they are well informed about the disorder stand to gain via psychoeducation, as it can reinforce their knowledge and help engender a sense of mastery and understanding of personal strengths and weaknesses. Further, information related to specific impacts of ADHD on functioning, as a college student, may be *especially* beneficial.

ADHD is often described as a disorder marked by three core symptoms: inattention (IA), hyperactivity, and impulsivity. The latter are together often abbreviated as HI. Inattention is marked by behaviors like *chronically* having difficulty following clearly delivered instructions, losing track of the topic in conversations, or being distracted by things in the environment that are not central to the task at hand. Hyperactivity-impulsivity is characterized by problems like *often* blurting out responses before a question has been fully posed, making decisions without adequately weighing the consequences (e.g., buying a car without figuring the total expense), and feelings of internal restlessness that may be manifested by chronic fidgeting. Emotional dysregulation is also more and more accepted as a central feature of ADHD (Barkley, 2015). This does not necessarily entail long periods of dysphoria, as is experienced in major depressive disorder, but instead is manifested as a *tendency* to react quickly and intensely to emotional stimuli. So, someone with ADHD who interprets a comment as an affront may seem to almost instantly become intensely angry, and to act accordingly (e.g., to curse the offending party and storm off). Such negative emotion does not necessarily last very long, but its immediate expression can be quite distracting and cause social problems, obviously, as well. Impairment related to the symptoms that are typical in ADHD extends across domains of living, including (a) school, (b) work, (c) family, peer, and romantic relations, (d) extracurricular (i.e., community-based) and sporting activities, (e) financial management, (f) driving, and (g) risky behaviors (e.g., higher accidental injury, unsafe sex, drug and alcohol use problems).

Historically, ADHD has been called various things (e.g., ADD, Hyperkinetic Disorder), but it has long been recognized as a discernable and impairing syndrome in children and adults. George Still, an English physician in the early 1900s, was the author of the first widely circulated and recognized description of ADHD, resulting from his presentations to the British Royal College of Physicians. However, a Scottish physician, Alexander Crichton, and a German counterpart, Melchior Weikard authored textbooks in the late 1700s that included disorders of attention that closely map onto our current definition of ADHD. One myth that your clients may have had to contend with is that ADHD is a disorder that was "invented" in a pharmacological and psychiatric industry

Table 1 Causal and probable exacerbating etiological factors of ADHD

Factors	Examples
Causal	
Genetics	Heritability of ADHD has been documented to be quite strong (estimated at .80), on par with schizophrenia. Specific genes involve dopamine and norepinephrine regulation (e.g., DRD4)
Other biological factors	Lead exposure, perinatal complications (e.g., oxygen deprivation), brain injury (e.g., TBI)
Probable exacerbating	
Nutrition	Children not eating breakfast have relatively poor concentration in school; limited intake of specific nutrients may impede brain function in executive areas
Sleep	Sleep loss is linked to impaired task adherence, inattention, emotional dysregulation
Stressors	Child or spouse abuse in the home is linked to impulsivity, inattention, and dysregulated emotion
Environment fit	Roles that demand effective multitasking and independent work will increase ADHD impairment; tasks that are inherently and frequently reinforcing (e.g., video games) will decrease apparent dysfunction

conspiracy (or something of the sort), but the historical study and documentation of ADHD-like conditions, far predates the advent of psychiatric medications in the 1950s and thereby renders such opinions practically invalid. Clients often find this information encouraging, and even self-affirming.

Over time, the etiology (i.e., the root causes and underlying mechanisms) of ADHD has been much researched. An adequate academic summary of this information would take far more space than could be allowed here, and the clinician is directed to the references noted earlier to develop a suitable foundation of knowledge. However, communication to the client regarding this topic can be relatively brief and focus on two aspects: (a) biological and genetic factors that predispose individuals to cognitive differences that can be deemed as *causes* of ADHD, and (b) environmental factors that *exacerbate* symptoms of ADHD. See Table 1 for an outline for presenting such information.

Another etiological constant has been an uneven distribution of ADHD across the sexes: ADHD occurs more frequently in males than it does in females. The male-to-female ratio was once thought to be as high as 10:1, but that was based on early studies concentrating on clinic samples. Epidemiological studies have put this ratio closer to 2:1 and indicate that girls and women tend to more predominantly experience inattention, as opposed to hyperactivity-impulsivity. Unfortunately, in practice, this has led to later identification of girls with ADHD, who may tend to be the "daydreamers" in elementary school but neither disrupt the class nor perform particularly well or poorly in academics, versus the boys who more commonly engage in behaviors like impulsive and maladaptive problem solving (e.g., pushing another student down to reach for an eraser instead of finding another) or hyperactivity (e.g., wandering into the hallway during a lesson) who tend to be referred for intervention.

A myth about ADHD that the therapist may want to dispel for clients, as it is a source of public disparagement of the disorder, is that ADHD occurs only in the United States. Cross-cultural studies have been conducted now on every continent in the world, and, while these have shown some variation in prevalence in children and adults across countries, the take-home message is clear: ADHD is a worldwide phenomenon.

Finally, we advise therapists to educate their clients regarding ADHD and its general, developmental course. While ADHD for most of the 20th century was assumed to be limited to children and adolescents, it has now been firmly established through longitudinal and epidemiological studies to persist into and even be identified initially in adulthood. This can look different depending on the individual. Some affected people exhibit many severely impairing symptoms and meet diagnostic criteria in childhood and adulthood. Others exhibit somewhat fewer symptoms as adults and may therefore only partially meet the diagnostic criteria yet *still* experience daily impairment related to those symptoms. Still others – note that this is a distinct minority – are affected adversely as children but either learn adaptive coping strategies, choose careers that do not require deskwork or sustained concentration, or simply "develop out" and do not experience meaningful ADHD-related impairment later in life. What is common across this spectrum is the presence of ADHD symptoms in childhood whether diagnosed earlier or later in life. *All* people with ADHD (or their parents or siblings, as the case may be) can point to behavioral markers in childhood of unusually elevated inattention and/or hyperactivity-impulsivity. For many, these symptoms persist across the entire lifespan.

What Are Executive Functioning Problems?

If there is a potential, common thread that links all the college students who may benefit most from the interventions outlined in this manual, it is what has come to be known as executive functioning problems. The definition of executive functioning (EF) has evolved over time, but EF has historically and neuropsychologically been linked to the prefrontal lobes of the cerebral cortex. Perhaps the most useful, global description of EF is that it encompasses several specific cognitive abilities related to *self-regulation*. These abilities include set-shifting (i.e., ability to purposefully shift attention back and forth between stimuli or tasks), working memory (i.e., taking in, using, and manipulating information in conscious mental awareness), and inhibition (i.e., the delay of automatic responses). Such abilities are the building blocks for cognitive behaviors such as planning and goal setting, completion of complex and effortful tasks, and successful social interactions. EF helps us to regulate our thoughts, feelings and behaviors, and to manage our time and resources. A student's ability to activate and apply EFs such as attention, judgment, planning, and behavioral regulation is important to academic and personal success.

As with most human characteristics, there is a natural range of ability in EF. On the high end of that range, one might envision a highly successful case manager working in a community-based clinic. From day to day, and hour to hour, she may see clients and must pay attention to and address their individual needs, shift gears quickly and focus to write succinct notes in between sessions, attend group staffing meetings and mentally weigh the benefits of commenting on other colleagues' cases, and inhibit the impulse to engage in off-task or socially inappropriate behavior (e.g., using a smartphone during a meeting). At the bottom end of the continuum, one might envision a high school student who is in behavioral and academic trouble. He could have a messy, disorganized room in which homework assignments (completed or not) are lost, chronically miss deadlines due to poor time management and planning, be unable to maintain focus and take appropriate notes in class, and impulsively yell or make crude gestures (or both) at peers, teachers, and parents who comment on any of these things, even with genuine intents to help.

While it is certain that some people in the general population have EF problems with no accompanying psychopathology, it is also the case that several—if not many—of the psychological disorders that are commonly classified and applicable to college students involve EF deficits. For example, individuals with mood and anxiety disorders characteristically exhibit concentration difficulties. Students who have learning disabilities may have more difficulty with accurate working memory. Those on the autism spectrum have difficulty inhibiting automatic behavior. However, perhaps the disorder that is most theorized to *hinge* upon dysfunctional EF is ADHD.

What Else Could be Causing Difficulty Concentrating?

Obviously, ADHD is by and large associated with chronic problems with attention and concentration. However, those with ADHD are not alone in having difficulty with attention and concentration. In fact, everyone has difficulty concentrating at times and we all have more difficulty concentrating on things we find less interesting. It may actually be more accurate to say that individuals with ADHD have difficulty *regulating attention* (e.g., noticing when attention shifts away from the current task and refocusing) than to say they have an attention deficit, since this latter term implies an inability to pay attention

(Barkley, 2015). Attentional capacity is likely on a continuum, and individuals with ADHD may need to be even more interested in something to pay attention to it. Furthermore, individuals with ADHD may become over-focused on things they find especially interesting (e.g., video games, action movies) and they may have difficulty switching their attention to something else once they become engaged.

As briefly noted above, there are other psychological disorders (and associated sub-threshold conditions) that may result in poor concentration, as well. For instance, distraction is one of the symptoms that is formally associated with major depressive disorder and persistent depressive disorder. Individuals with anxiety disorders who are in the presence of their feared stimulus (e.g., being in a discussion-based seminar while having Social Anxiety Disorder) also appear to suffer from poor concentration to tasks.

Attention has recently been drawn to a cluster of symptoms that pertains directly to one's ability to focus and varies independently from ADHD, which has been traditionally referred to as *sluggish cognitive tempo* but more recently as concentration deficit disorder (CDD; Barkley, 2014). While CDD has relatively few supporters, to date, for inclusion as a formal diagnostic category, converging evidence suggests two cognitive-behavioral symptomatic dimensions (i.e., day-dreamy, sluggish-underactive) that are largely associated with social impairment (i.e., isolation), although some newer evidence suggests it poses difficulties in academics, as well.

Environmental issues have been implicated in acute concentration difficulties, as well. Clearly, the presence of a tangible and intense stressor (e.g., living in a new town and college setting) can increase anxiety, lead to cognitive preoccupations, and distract individuals from daily academic or living tasks that college students need to complete. There are a vast variety of stressors that could have this effect, and individuals will have differing levels of stress sensitivity and coping skills that can influence their adjustment, as well. As also noted above in exacerbating factors for ADHD, sleep debt (i.e., chronic sleep latency or interruption associated with less-than-optimal sleep time) and poor nutrition (i.e., either lack of adequate caloric or nutrient intake) can be associated with diminished attentional capacity, as well.

Finally, there are a range of medical and physical conditions that could contribute to problems with concentration and attention. These include hypoglycemia, allergies, thyroid problems, anemia, diabetes, and cardiovascular (i.e., heart) disease. As such, adequate and regular screening by a medical professional should be a routine part of all adults' lives (including college students), and a lack of follow-through in this area is cause for change, especially for any who have a family history that includes these or related conditions.

Due to these and other potential confounds in the *source* of concentration difficulties, it is quite important as a therapist to ensure that this has received sufficient consideration in case conceptualization. Psychoeducation regarding these factors influencing attention and concentration would productively be paired with discussion regarding whether students view the same as problematic in their current lives, and what steps (if any) that would be beyond the scope of the interventions in this manual are warranted (e.g., obtaining a physical for a student who has not had one recently, obtaining a nutritional consultation).

How Is ADHD Assessed?

An evidence-based assessment of ADHD in a college student or adult consists of multiple components. First, the clinician should recommend a medical eva-luation to rule out any physical problems as a cause of their symptoms. This can often be conducted through student health services available at many institutions. Next, the clinician should collect self-report rating scales from the client regarding their childhood and current behavior. This should include ADHD symptoms (e.g., BAARS) as well as impairment rating scales (e.g., WFIRS). Furthermore, it is critically important that the clinician collect collateral report rating scales regarding the client's childhood and current behavior (i.e., ADHD symptoms and impairment). For childhood behavior, the optimal collateral reporter might be a parent or a sibling. For current behavior, the optimal reporter might be a significant other, a close friend, a roommate, or a parent. Thus, one parent might be able to complete both the collateral childhood and current behavior reports, and this may be the most efficient strategy for col-lecting this information. It is important to have a discussion with the client about who the optimal collateral reporters might be. We want to ensure these reporters are individuals who have been exposed to the client's behavior in a variety of situations (e.g., academic, domestic, interpersonal). In some cases, the client may have reservations about asking certain individuals to complete these rating scales. For example, he or she may have a parent who does not "believe" in ADHD or psychological disorders and, thus, may be reluctant to ask a parent to complete these rating scales. Although this is understandable, it could un-dermine the clinician's ability to reach a diagnostic conclusion since evidence of several childhood symptoms is necessary for a diagnosis. Clients should be discouraged from asking less than optimal reporters (i.e., those who do not have as much information about their behavior) to complete these rating scales as the information obtained may not be valid.

Following the completion of self- and other report rating scales, the assessing clinician should conduct a structured or semi-structured diagnostic interview with the client. This interview should include ADHD symptoms as well as other possible comorbid issues (e.g., depression, anxiety, substance use disorders, eating disorders). Next, it is typically recommended that cognitive and achievement testing be conducted to rule out developmental delays as well as comorbid learning disorders. In our clinical experience, we have found that this is not always feasible given a lack of resources. We often have long waitlists in our psychology clinics for ADHD assessments, and we have found that the inclusion of cognitive and achievement testing is not as critical as it is with children for a couple of reasons. First, college students are unlikely to have cognitive abilities that are extremely low given that they have graduated from high school and been admitted to college. Second, even if comorbid learning disorders exist, the interventions are much more limited at this age than in childhood. Thus, we recommend completing cognitive and achievement testing *if* you have the resources *and* the client would like to rule out comorbid learning problems.

In assessment for ADHD, it is sometimes recommended that the clinician administer a continuous performance task (CPT) to the client. It is important to note that while these tests cannot be used to rule in or rule out ADHD due to a high rate of false positives, it can be helpful to have one more piece of information to examine along with the results of rating scales and clinical interviews. In addition, CPTs are thought to be a reasonable safeguard against malingering. In our experience, college students who do not have ADHD and are medication-seeking often score even lower than the typical individual with ADHD.

All of the information collected should be considered when making diagnostic conclusions regarding an ADHD diagnosis.

General Discussion

The following is a list of possible discussion questions, all appropriate for groups or individuals:

1 When were you first diagnosed with ADHD? Describe your experience with being diagnosed with ADHD.
2 Did you receive an evidence-based assessment?
3 Have you received medication or therapy treatment in the past?
4 Why did you decide to seek treatment now?
5 What do you hope to gain from treatment? What are your goals or expected outcomes?

Facilitate discussion for the rest of the session, centering around these or other questions and topics that arise that are pertinent to knowing more about ADHD and/or participant(s) expression of their experiences.

Discuss Homework and Schedule Next Session

For homework, students should obtain copies of any previous psychological assessment(s) and bring these with them to the next session. That session should be scheduled with the client(s) at this point.

References

Barkley, R.A. (Ed.). (2015). *Attention-deficit hyperactivity disorder: A handbook for diagnosis and treatment* (4th ed.). The Guilford Press.

Barkley, R.A., Murphy, K.R., & Fischer, M. (2008). *ADHD in adults: What the science says.* Guilford Press.

Barkley, R.A. (2014). Sluggish cognitive tempo (concentration deficit disorder?): Current status, future directions, and a plea to change the name. *Journal of Abnormal Child Psychology, 42*(1), 117–125. 10.1007/s10802-013-9824-y

Chew, B.L., Jensen, S.A., & Rosén, L.A. (2009). College students' attitudes toward their ADHD peers. *Journal of Attention Disorders, 13*(3), 271–276. 10.1177/1087054709333347

Hallowell, E.M. & Ratey, J.J. (2011). *Driven to distraction: Recognizing and coping with attention deficit disorder from childhood through adulthood.* Anchor Books.

Session 2: Psychosocial and Medication Treatments for ADHD

Session Outline

1 Check-in with client(s)
2 Set agenda
3 How is ADHD treated?
4 Are psychosocial interventions or psychotherapy effective for college students with ADHD?
5 Is medication treatment effective for college students with ADHD?
6 What should college students with ADHD know about stimulant medication for ADHD?
7 General discussion
8 Discuss homework
9 Schedule next session

Session Organization

Administration Format

Session 2 can be administered in a group or individual format. As in Session 1, however, a group session has advantages; students often benefit from sharing their struggles with ADHD and related impairment, and a group is more efficient in that it educates several clients at once. In addition to providing the opportunity for support, encouragement, and modeling, research suggests that clients who interact with others who have ADHD have reduced stigma toward ADHD (Chew, Jensen & Rosen, 2009). Nonetheless, an individual session is acceptable if a group session is not indicated or practical.

Materials Needed

The therapist should have a whiteboard, flipchart, or a projected digital document to capture group ideas and/or present material.

DOI: 10.4324/9781003149590-4

- A list of "take home messages" regarding the session's content as well as instructions/goals for at-home work prior to the next session are also useful to give to clients as references.

Session Content

Check-in with Client(s)

Check-in time can be used to solicit brief discussion, or simply to see how things are going and build rapport. If this session is the first meeting with the client(s), check-in might focus more on feelings and expectations about therapy. In the event that you have completed Educating Clients Session 1 with your client(s), check-in may focus on discussion of what they learned in going back through their latest psychological assessment report (e.g., perspective gained on the assessment itself). In any case, aim for this to be brief (< 5 minutes), encouraging for any additional discussion of this sort to be postponed until after the session content is completed. See therapist-client check-in dialog example in Skill 1: Session 1 as a model for this interaction, if needed. We also recommend having your client complete the *Progress Tracker* (see Appendix B), and briefly touching base on any declines or improvements in school functioning.

Set Agenda

Introduce the agenda for this session to the client (see above). It may be helpful to have a visual aid to refer to, such as a flip chart or projected PowerPoint slide or printed handout. At this time it might also be helpful to remind clients to write notes regarding important points in a therapy notebook. Setting the agenda should be speedily completed (< 2 minutes). See therapist-client agenda-setting dialog example in Skill 1: Session 1 as a model, if needed.

How Is ADHD Treated?

In children, there is substantial research support for treating ADHD with a combination of behavioral management and medication treatment (Evans, Owens & Bunford, 2014). Behavioral management includes behavioral parent training and behavioral classroom management. Medication treatment includes stimulant and non-stimulant interventions, but stimulants are by far the most prescribed.

Regarding treating ADHD in adolescents (ages 13–17), emerging adults (ages 18–25), and adults (ages 26 and up), much less research has been conducted. However, a few things are clear. First, while adolescents appear to have more varied responses to stimulant medications than do children (e.g., Molina et al., 2009), there is very scant data to draw on regarding treatment response in adults. However, available data suggests that these stimulants do tend to have at least short-term efficacy at addressing ADHD-related problems (Fredriksen et al., 2013) in college students (DuPaul et al., 2012) and mature adults, alike (Faraone et al., 2004; Lensing et al., 2014; Weyandt et al., 2014). Second, behavioral management via parents and teachers is less applicable for adolescents and not relevant for adults. Therefore, many of the interventions that are being evaluated for the treatment of ADHD in adolescents and adults fall into a category that has been referred to as training interventions (Evans et al., 2014). Whereas behavior management involves training parents and teachers to change a child's behavior by modifying contingencies in the child's environment (e.g., rewards and punishments), training interventions involve providing skills training to individuals who then use them independently.

Are Psychosocial Interventions or Psychotherapy Effective for College Students with ADHD?

There are currently only a handful of published studies examining the effectiveness of psychosocial interventions for ADHD in college students (e.g., Eddy et al., 2015; Hartung et al., 2022; LaCount et al., 2015; Anastopoulos & King, 2015). Research with adolescents, and adults beyond college age, has relevance for this age group but there are also some unique issues for college students. Compared to high school students, college students face greater academic demands in a setting with less structure and more distractions. Moreover, adults beyond college age are typically not engaged in academic pursuits. For these reasons, more research is needed to examine the effectiveness of psychosocial treatments specifically for college students.

Taken together, the existing studies provide preliminary support for a variety of cognitive and behavioral intervention strategies including: (a) psychoeducation, (b) organization, time management and planning training (OTMP), (c) study skills training, and (d) adaptive thinking or cognitive restructuring. Further, recent research suggests that the delivery of such interventions via internet-based modalities may be a viable, effective option, as compared to face-to-face therapy (Pettersson et al., 2014), which may be especially relevant to college populations and merits further investigation. However, it should be noted that these intervention strategies have been studied in varying packages and dismantling studies have only recently begun to examine whether these strategies are most effective when provided individually or collectively (e.g., LaCount et al., 2018).

In addition to dismantling studies of such "mainline" CBT interventions for adults, other specific strategies that borrow-from or are based on cognitive-behavioral principles have shown some efficacy at addressing ADHD-related problems and bear consideration here. Mindfulness meditation techniques have been shown in open and pilot trials to be promising interventions, resulting in self-reported and, to a lesser extent, clinician-rated improvements in core

ADHD symptoms, executive functioning, and comorbid anxiety and depression (Edel et al., 2017; Mitchell et al., 2017; Zylowska et al., 2008). Fleming and colleagues (Fleming et al., 2015) implemented a dialectical behavior therapy (DBT) protocol specifically tailored to the needs of college students with ADHD in a randomized trial, emphasizing adaptive, emotional regulation and problem-solving skills and found the DBT intervention to be effective at reducing reported ADHD symptoms and, to a lesser degree, improving quality of life.

Is Medication Treatment Effective for College Students with ADHD?

Currently, there is only one published study of the effectiveness of medication for the treatment of ADHD in college students (i.e., DuPaul et al., 2012). As mentioned previously, research with adolescents and adults may be relevant for college students but this group also has some unique developmental and environmental issues. Furthermore, there are also concerns about the dispersion of stimulant medication on college campuses (Hartung et al., 2013). For these reasons, more research is needed to examine the effectiveness of medication treatments specifically for college students.

Medication treatment of ADHD involves stimulants and non-stimulants. Central nervous system (CNS) stimulants are considered a first-line treatment for ADHD, given the wealth of research on their effectiveness and safety (Fredriksen et al., 2013). The most used stimulants for ADHD are those in the methylphenidate (e.g., Ritalin, Focalin, Concerta) and the amphetamine (e.g., Adderall, Vyvanse) families (Huang & Tsai, 2011). Non-stimulants have been shown to be effective to a lesser degree than the stimulants and are newer to the market, and are, therefore, prescribed less frequently (Huang & Tsai, 2011). The most used and studied non-stimulant is atomoxetine (i.e., Strattera), with antidepressants just beginning to be empirically examined for ADHD treatment (e.g., duloxetine, marketed as Cymbalta; Bilodeau et al., 2014). While atomoxetine is not quite as effective as stimulant medications at addressing core symptoms of ADHD, it has a longer half-life and as such is continuously effective, whereas stimulants are short acting with effects lasting 4 to 12 hours depending on the formulation. Furthermore, atomoxetine has less abuse potential because it is not fully effective unless taken regularly. There is a wealth of research on stimulant treatment of ADHD in children that demonstrates that these medications are highly effective for about 70% of children with ADHD who are classified as *responders* (Pelham, Wheeler, & Chronis, 1998). The magnitude of the effect is one of the largest seen in the treatment of mental health disorders (Spencer et al., 2000). There is much less research on the effectiveness of these medications with adults. As noted already, there is only one published study on the effectiveness of a stimulant in college students, which we will review next (DuPaul et al., 2012). In sum, the research on the use of stimulants in adults suggest (a) that these groups tend to respond less consistently, (b) experience more side effects, and as a result, (c) take stimulant medications less consistently than children who are supervised by parents (Prince et al., 2015).

Given that stimulant medications have the most support for the treatment of ADHD in other age groups, research should begin with this class of medications for college students with ADHD. DuPaul et al. (2012) examined the effectiveness of Lisdexamfetamine Dimesylate (i.e., Vyvanse), which is a stimulant, in college students. They found significant improvements for college students taking this medication in terms of ADHD symptoms and executive functioning. Nonetheless, improvements in these areas for college students with ADHD did not bring their levels of functioning into the range that was comparable to typical peers. As such, this stimulant medication has potential for the treatment of ADHD, but psychosocial interventions are also needed. Furthermore, the authors did not assess the impact of medication use on long-term academic performance. Therefore, additional research is needed to determine whether stimulant medication and/or psychosocial treatments will result in improved academic performance for college students with ADHD.

While it should be evident from even this summary that there is not a shortage of *options* for college students to pursue in terms of treating ADHD, it must be noted that there are significant barriers to attaining such treatment. For many college students, the most viable provider of mental health interventions, regarding both cost and convenience, is their institution's health (i.e., medical) services departments and counseling centers. Recent research derived from a national sample of counseling center directors and physicians and nurses in university health services indicates these front-line professionals perceive ADHD in college students to be difficult to diagnose and recognize, and that referral to private or community-based providers is the most common response when ADHD is suspected (Thomas et al., 2014). It may be that the comorbid symptoms that often exist in college students with ADHD (e.g., anxiety, depression, stress, low self-worth) make it harder to recognize inattention as a contributing factor, especially since difficulty concentrating is also seen in those with anxiety and/or depression. Furthermore, comprehensive psychological assessment typically does not occur in student health or university counseling centers due to time constraints and resource limitations. This situation may leave many affected students in a lurch, without the transportation, time, or financial resources to pursue effective assessment and intervention.

What Should College Students with ADHD Know about Stimulant Medication Treatments for ADHD?

First, as discussed previously, college students should be aware that these medications have been shown to be effective for the treatment of ADHD in children, adolescents, and adults with ADHD. In addition, one recent study has extended this evidence to college students (DuPaul et al., 2012).

Second, students should be aware that not everyone has a positive response to these medications and an individual's response to one stimulant may be different than their response to another stimulant. A positive response includes: (a) the desired clinical response of improved attention and concentration and/ or decreased hyperactivity and impulsivity and (b) a lack of intolerable side effects (e.g., difficulty sleeping, increased anxiety, increased emotionality, sleep difficulty, and decreased appetite). Students may need to experiment, under the supervision of their prescribing physician, with multiple stimulants before finding one that is optimal in terms of clinical response and side effects. Typically, it recommended that one type of stimulant be tried first (i.e., one from the methylphenidate family or one from the amphetamine family). If the response is not optimal, it is recommended that the other type of stimulant be tried next (Prince et al., 2015).

Although these medications are quite safe when taken as prescribed, they should only be taken by individuals who have been: (a) diagnosed with ADHD via an evidence-based assessment including collateral rating scales; (b) examined by a physician to rule out cardiovascular problems or other health-related issues that might impact the safety of stimulants; and (c) received a prescription from a medical provider. Furthermore, clients should be encouraged to actively interact with their psychiatrist or primary-care physician to make sure that they are taking the optimal stimulant medication, at the appropriate frequency. Based on our clinical experience, it appears that it is fairly common for college students to have a prescription for a stimulant medication that they do not experience as optimal. In such cases, we think it is important to help clients decide if they want to discontinue medication treatment or talk with their physician about a change in dose or prescription of another stimulant (or non-stimulant). For example, a student client who has a less than optimal response to a stimulant of one variety (e.g., methylphenidate family) may want to ask their prescriber about trying another type of stimulant (e.g., amphetamine family). It is certainly common for individuals to respond differently to the various stimulants. Therefore, if one stimulant is effective but creates unwanted side effects for an individual, this does not mean that this individual will respond to all the stimulants in this same way. Thus, student clients may need to try several stimulants, under medical supervision, before finding the optimal formulation and dose. The therapist is encouraged to keep in mind that students who are not experiencing meaningful benefit from their prescriptions may be more likely to have extra pills, as they may not take their medication regularly. In such cases, students should always be reminded not to share any extra pills with friends or acquaintances, as we will discuss in more detail below.

Third, students should know that these medications are short-acting and, therefore, they will not help the student manage his or her symptoms all the time. For example, a student who has a positive response to a stimulant may still have difficulty with her morning routine and getting to class on time because her medication, which she took with breakfast, has not yet reached its full effect. Further, some students have reported that stimulant medications help them concentrate for longer periods of time, but they do not help as much with organization and time management. Thus, a student may be able to study for longer periods of time but still might not be successful at organizing long-term projects or prioritizing tasks. This is one reason stimulant medications may be most optimal when used in combination with psychosocial treatments (e.g., organizational training, study skills training).

Fourth, students should know that stimulants are a safe and effective treatment for ADHD and minimal long-term side effects have been identified (Craig et al., 2015). Nonetheless, research on the "long-term" outcomes has not extended beyond a two-year period of use. In sum, there do not appear to be significant long-term side effects associated with use of stimulant medications for two years or less, but there is not yet empirical data to conclude that longer use is equally safe.

Last, but not least, students should know that it is unsafe and illegal to sell, or even share, stimulant medications. College students should be informed that a person who does not have a prescription should not take these medications due to unknown health risks. Specifically, there have been a small number of cases involving individuals who had known or unknown cardiovascular problems and experienced sudden death in response to stimulant medications. Thus, stimulant medications are not recommended for individuals with cardiovascular problems. Hartung et al. (2013) reported that 81% of college students who misused stimulants by taking them without a prescription obtained them from a friend. Thus, the legal, ethical, and health-related risks of sharing stimulant medications with a friend do not appear widely understood by college students and this information needs to be clearly conveyed by medical providers and reiterated by therapists.

General Discussion

At this point, clients have heard a lot about treatment for ADHD. Some may want to learn more specifics, and others may have questions about topics that were not covered. Allow a little time for discussion at this point; if clients still have questions or you need to research or find related answers, make sure to follow up after the session is completed.

Discuss Homework and Schedule Next Meeting

Students should find out if they have received any treatments for ADHD in the past and whether the treatments were effective. This will involve having conversations with parents or other relatives (e.g., siblings, aunts, uncles, and grandparents). Also, students who are currently taking medication for ADHD should report the name of the medication, dosage, frequency/regularity of use, and perceived effectiveness to their therapist at the next session. That session should be scheduled with the client(s) at this point.

References

Anastopoulos, A.D., & King, K.A. (2015). A cognitive-behavior therapy and mentoring program for college students with ADHD. *Cognitive and Behavioral Practice, 22*(2), 141–151. 10.1016/j.cbpra.2014.01.002

Bilodeau, M., Simon, T., Beauchamp, M.H., Lespérance, P., Dubreucq, S., Dorée, J.P., & Tourjman, S.V. (2014). Duloxetine in adults with ADHD: A randomized, placebo-controlled pilot study. *Journal of Attention Disorders, 18*(2), 169–175. 10.1177/1087054 712443157

Chew, B.L., Jensen, S.A., & Rosén, L.A. (2009). College students' attitudes toward their ADHD peers. *Journal of Attention Disorders, 13*(3), 271–276. 10.1177/1087054 709333347

Craig, S.G., Davies, G., Schibuk, L., Weiss, M.D., & Hetchman, L. (2015). Long-term effects of stimulant treatment for ADHD: What can we tell our patients? *Current Developmental Disorders Reports, 2*, 1–9.

Dupaul, G.J., Weyandt, L.L., Rossi, J.S., Vilardo, B.A., O'Dell, S.M., Carson, K.M., Verdi, G., & Swentosky, A. (2012). Double-blind, placebo-controlled, crossover study of the efficacy and safety of lisdexamfetamine dimesylate in college students with ADHD. *Journal of Attention Disorders, 16*(3), 202–220. 10.1177/1087054711427299

Eddy, L.D., Canu, W.H., Broman-Fulks, J.J., & Michael, K.D. (2015). Brief cognitive behavioral therapy for college students with ADHD: A case series report. *Cognitive and Behavioral Practice, 22*(2), 127–140. 10.1016/j.cbpra.2014.05.005

Edel, M.A., Hölter, T., Wassink, K., & Juckel, G. (2017). A comparison of mindfulness-based group training and skills group training in adults with ADHD. *Journal of Attention Disorders, 21*(6), 533–539. 10.1177/1087054714551635

Evans, S.W., Owens, J.S., & Bunford, N. (2014). Evidence-based psychosocial treatments for children and adolescents with attention-deficit/hyperactivity disorder. *Journal of Clinical Child and Adolescent Psychology, 43*(4), 527–551. 10.1080/15374416. 2013.850700

Faraone, S.V., Spencer, T., Aleardi, M., Pagano, C., & Biederman, J. (2004). Meta-analysis of the efficacy of methylphenidate for treating adult attention-deficit/hyperactivity disorder. *Journal of Clinical Psychopharmacology, 24*(1), 24–29. 10.1097/01. jcp.0000108984.11879.95

Fleming, A.P., McMahon, R.J., Moran, L.R., Peterson, A.P., & Dreessen, A. (2015). Pilot randomized controlled trial of dialectical behavior therapy group skills training for

ADHD among college students. *Journal of Attention Disorders*, *19*(3), 260–271. 10.1177/1087054714535951

Fredriksen, M., Halmøy, A., Faraone, S.V., & Haavik, J. (2013). Long-term efficacy and safety of treatment with stimulants and atomoxetine in adult ADHD: A review of controlled and naturalistic studies. *European Neuropsychopharmacology: The Journal of the European College of Neuropsychopharmacology*, *23*(6), 508–527. 10.1016/j.euroneuro.2012.07.016

Hartung, C.M., Canu, W.H., Cleveland, C.S., Lefler, E.K., Mignogna, M.J., Fedele, D.A., Correia, C.J., Leffingwell, T.R., & Clapp, J.D. (2013). Stimulant medication use in college students: comparison of appropriate users, misusers, and nonusers. *Psychology of Addictive Behaviors: Journal of the Society of Psychologists in Addictive Behaviors*, *27*(3), 832–840. 10.1037/a0033822

Hartung, C.M., Canu, W.H., Serrano, J.W., Vasko, J.M., Stevens, A.E., Abu-Ramadan, T.M., Bodalski, E.A., Neger, E.N., Bridges, R.M., Gleason, L.L., Anzalone, C., & Flory, K. (2022). A new organizational and study skills intervention for college students with ADHD. *Cognitive and Behavioral Practice*, *29*(2), 411–424. 10.1016/j.cbpra.2020.09.005

Huang, Y.S., & Tsai, M.H. (2011). Long-term outcomes with medications for attention-deficit hyperactivity disorder: Current status of knowledge. *CNS Drugs*, *25*(7), 539–554. 10.2165/11589380-000000000-00000

LaCount, P.A., Hartung, C.M., Shelton, C.R., Clapp, J.D., & Clapp, T.K.W. (2015). Preliminary evaluation of a combined group and individual treatment for college students with attention-deficit/hyperactivity disorder. *Cognitive and Behavioral Practice*, *22*(2), 152–160. 10.1016/j.cbpra.2014.07.004

LaCount, P.A., Hartung, C.M., Shelton, C.R., & Stevens, A.E. (2018). Efficacy of an organizational skills intervention for college students with ADHD symptomatology and academic difficulties. *Journal of Attention Disorders*, *22*, 356–367. 10.1177/1087054715594423

Lensing, M.B., Zeiner, P., Sandvik, L., & Opjordsmoen, S. (2014). Psychopharmacological treatment of ADHD in adults aged 50+: An empirical study. *Journal of Attention Disorders*, *19*(5), 380–389. 10.1177/1087054714527342

Mitchell, J.T., McIntyre, E.M., English, J.S., Dennis, M.F., Beckham, J.C., & Kollins, S.H. (2017). A pilot trial of mindfulness meditation training for ADHD in adulthood: Impact on core symptoms, executive functioning, and emotion dysregulation. *Journal of Attention Disorders*, *21* (13), 1105–1120. 10.1177/1087054713513328

Molina, B., Hinshaw, S.P., Swanson, J.M., Arnold, L.E., Vitiello, B., Jensen, P.S., Epstein, J.N., Hoza, B., Hechtman, L., Abikoff, H.B., Elliott, G.R., Greenhill, L.L., Newcorn, J.H., Wells, K.C., Wigal, T., Gibbons, R.D., Hur, K., Houck, P.R., & MTA Cooperative Group (2009). The MTA at 8 years: prospective follow-up of children treated for combined-type ADHD in a multisite study. *Journal of the American Academy of Child and Adolescent Psychiatry*, *48*(5), 484–500. 10.1097/CHI.0b013e31819c23d0

Pelham, W.E., Jr, Wheeler, T., & Chronis, A. (1998). Empirically supported psychosocial treatments for attention deficit hyperactivity disorder. *Journal of Clinical Child Psychology*, *27*(2), 190–205. 10.1207/s15374424jccp2702_6

Pettersson, R., Söderström, S., Edlund-Söderström, K., & Nilsson, K.W. (2014). Internet-based cognitive behavioral therapy for adults With ADHD in outpatient psychiatric care. *Journal of Attention Disorders, 21*(6), 508–521. 10.1177/1087054714539998

Prince, J.B., Wilens, T.E., Spencer, T.J., & Biederman, J. (2015). Pharmacotherapy of ADHD in adults. In R.A. Barkley (Ed.), *Attention-Deficit Hyperactivity Disorder: A Handbook for Diagnosis and Treatment* (pp. 826–860). The Guilford Press.

Spencer, T., Biederman, J., & Wilens, T. (2000). Pharmacotherapy of attention deficit hyperactivity disorder. *Child and Adolescent Psychiatric Clinics of North America, 9,* 77–97.

Thomas, M., Rostain, A., Corso, R., Babcock, T., & Madhoo, M. (2014). ADHD in the college setting: Current perceptions and future vision. *Journal of Attention Disorders, 19*(8), 643–654. 10.1177/1087054714527789

Weyandt, L.L., Oster, D.R., Marraccini, M.E., Gudmundsdottir, B.G., Munro, B.A., Zavras, B.M., & Kuhar, B. (2014). Pharmacological interventions for adolescents and adults with ADHD: Stimulant and nonstimulant medications and misuse of prescription stimulants. *Psychology Research and Behavior Management, 7,* 223–249. 10.2147/PRBM.S47013

Zylowska, L., Ackerman, D.L., Yang, M.H., Futrell, J.L., Horton, N.L., Hale, T.S., Pataki, C., & Smalley, S.L. (2008). Mindfulness meditation training in adults and adolescents with ADHD: A feasibility study. *Journal of Attention Disorders, 11*(6), 737–746. 10.1177/1087054707308502

Skill 1: Organization, Time Management, and Planning Skills

(~4 sessions)

Corresponds to Skillset 1 in the *Thriving in College* Student Workbook

Background for the Therapist

Organization, time management and planning (OTMP) skills are essential for success in both college and professional careers. These skills, which include effective use of personal planners, task lists, and prioritization techniques, have typically been self-taught or learned through trial-and-error, and are useful to all adults but especially to individuals who have more difficulty with OTMP skills, such as those with ADHD. This may be particularly true for college students with ADHD, who must balance their new responsibilities and expectations of independence in learning and life in the context of OTMP deficits. Mental health researchers and professionals have begun to explicitly teach these skills to adolescents and adults with ADHD as one component of intervention to reduce maladjustment. The sooner such skills are integrated into daily life, the greater the benefit. For instance, adolescents in middle or high school who struggle academically yet learn, and effectively implement, OTMP skills will not only be more likely to perform satisfactorily in their current academic work but will also be ahead of peers without such intervention regarding adapting to more demanding work of subsequent grades and even vocations.

Inherently, the most important "job" of college students is to learn and, relatedly, to earn passing grades. Consequently, a primary goal of teaching OTMP skills to this population is to optimize academic performance (e.g., bolster GPA and decrease number of course withdrawals). OTMP skills can help in this way by providing structure for students to keep track of when assignments are due and when exams will be given so they can choose how to best allocate their time and energy. OTMP can also be used to help overcome negative motivation for tackling more complex assignments (e.g., term papers). This can be accomplished by parceling tasks and subtasks that are necessary for completion of a complex assignment into manageable chunks whose sequential completion provides a steady flow of reinforcement. While there may be several

DOI: 10.4324/9781003149590-5

other strategies that could provide some additional benefit, a very concise set of strategies that we have found to provide significant adaptive improvement for college students is:

- Adopt and consistently use a *calendar and task or to-do list system*
- Systematically *prioritize tasks* based on urgency and importance
- *Break tasks into smaller steps* to prevent procrastination and increase satisfaction
- *Reward yourself* for completing tasks using the when-then principle

As outlined in this module, these skills can be presented to students in a group, individual or combined individual-and-group therapy format. We recommend that these OTMP skills be introduced and practiced during four-to-five therapy sessions and that they be seen, along with psychoeducation (i.e., Educating Clients module), as **core elements of standard CBT intervention for college students with ADHD or other learning challenges**.

Assessing Baseline OTMP Skills

As noted in this manual's introduction, and as with any intervention to strengthen adaptive behavior, it is important to verify that clients *have* deficits in organization, time management, and/or planning before proceeding. For instance, it might be

---

Box 1 Items to use for progress tracking in treatment

1. I have difficulty with attendance or being late at school or work.
2. I have difficulty keeping appointments (doctor, professor, etc.,).
3. I have trouble keeping track of when tests are scheduled or when assignments are due.
4. I have difficulty getting to bed at a reasonable time.
5. I have problems getting ready to leave for the day.
6. Others do important things for me (parents, friends, roommates, etc.,).
7. I have problems getting work done efficiently (completing assignments, etc.,).
8. I have problems getting started on tasks at school and/or work.
9. I have problems working to my potential (assignments are rushed or missing, etc.,).
10. I use the internet, social media, video games, or TV excessively or inappropriately.
11. I have problems keeping up with chores (laundry, dishes, shopping, etc.,).
12. I have problems managing money (paying bills on time, sticking to my budget, etc.,).

that a client is effectively using a planner to keep track of upcoming commitments, appointments, and tasks, but failing miserably at prioritizing work on important, long-term projects. The first step, of course, is to talk with your client during an individual intake about OTMP and to get a sense for how consistently and effectively they are using the related skills already. In Box 1, we list the items and response scale we suggest for assessing OTMP skills throughout the course of treatment. We have used this OTMP scale to assess skill usage in our own research, and provide an easy-to-use form for your use in Appendix B (i.e., *Progress Tracker*). We recommend using this or an alternative measure to assess OTMP skills at the outset of therapy and to track progress over time.

In addition to these measures, there are other standardized measures you could consider using to gain further information about the importance of and direction for OTMP training for any individual client. For instance, the *Learning and Study Strategies Inventory* (LASSI; Weinstein & Palmer, 2002), which provides comprehensive information related to academic preparation and skills and potentially important insights for treatment planning and outcome assessment, includes a *Time Management Scale* that relates to OTMP in the college setting. A few other instruments that you might wish to consider employing for assessment of baseline OTMP abilities are provided in Appendix B.

Student Workbook

If you are using the *Thriving in College* student workbook, you will find that Skillset 1 on *Organization and Time Management* corresponds to the material in this section. The following chart provides more information on which individual modules in the workbook correspond to each session in this section.

Therapist Guide Session	Workbook Modules
1	1.0 Why it Matters, Pre-Assessment, & Roadmap
	1.1 Choose Your Personal Calendar and Task List
2	1.2 How to Use Your Calendar and Task List Effectively
3	1.3 Set Your Priorities
	1.4 Make Yourself Do Things
4	1.5 Getting Unstuck from Procrastination

Reference

Weinstein, C.E. & Palmer, D.R. (2002). *Learning and study strategies inventory (LASSI): Users manual.* H & H Publishing.

Session 1: Choosing a Calendar and Task List System

Corresponds to Modules 1.0 and 1.1 in the *Thriving in College* Student Workbook

Session Outline

1 Check-in with client(s)
2 Set agenda
3 Discuss why organizational skills are so important for people with ADHD
4 Administer assessments of OTMP skills
5 Choosing a calendar system
6 Choosing a task list system
7 Discuss homework
8 Set time and date for the next meeting

Session Organization

Administration Format

Session 1 can be administered in a group or individual format. A group session is optimal because students often benefit from sharing their struggles and successes with using calendars and task list systems and helping each other in troubleshooting that process. However, an individual session is acceptable if a group session is not indicated or practical.

Materials Needed

The therapist should bring a whiteboard, flipchart, or projected document to capture group ideas. The therapist is also encouraged to bring several examples of adequate calendar systems to the session to illustrate potentially notable features. The latter includes (a) adequate space to record both scheduled meetings and daily tasks, (b) adequate chronological span (i.e., ability to plan at least one semester), and (c) portability and accessibility (e.g., electronic calendars are handy on iPhones and Android devices). Further, student clients should be told to bring a notebook or laptop to every session in this module to facilitate the taking of notes, which is vital to the retention of information and the use thereof between sessions. Therapists might

DOI: 10.4324/9781003149590-6

productively display a list of "take home messages" at the end of each session to make sure that clients record key concepts and directions for intersession work. The therapist should also bring enough copies of the OTMP self-reports scales (see Appendix B) so that the client(s) can complete this impairment inventory during the session.

Session Content

Check in with client(s)

It is likely that clients have recently completed the psychoeducation module of this intervention (i.e., Educating Clients), and as such may have questions or comments regarding that material. Check-in time can be used to solicit brief discussion, or simply to see how things are going and build rapport (see Dialogue 1 for an example). If this session is the first meeting with clients, check-in might focus more on feelings and expectations about therapy. In any event, aim for this to be brief (<5 minutes), encouraging for any additional discussion of this sort to be postponed until after the session content is completed. We also recommend having your client complete the *Progress Tracker* (see Appendix B), and briefly touching base on any declines or improvements in school functioning.

Dialogue 1

Therapist: *Welcome back. I am eager to talk about this session's content about organization skills because I think this is something that most people with ADHD can benefit from. However, I want to take a few minutes to check in with you first. Is there anything that you have been wondering about since the last time we met? Or maybe you have questions or thoughts about how your therapy will progress from here?*

Client: *Well, not really any questions. I think I understand ADHD a lot better, and was talking with my mom about it, and there were things that she didn't know that I learned about. It felt good, like I'm finally taking charge of this for myself. I am looking forward to learning more.*

Therapist: *That's great! Let's begin, then.*

Note: If clients have questions or comments about prior material regarding ADHD, try to answer these concisely, but if they are bigger topics, make note of these now and address these with clients at the end of the session or via readings and other resources.

Set agenda

Introduce the agenda for this session to the client (see Dialogue 2). It may be helpful to have a visual aid to refer to, such as a flip chart or projected PowerPoint slide or printed handout. At this time, it might also be helpful to remind clients to write notes regarding important points in a therapy notebook. Setting the agenda should be speedily completed (< 2 minutes).

Dialogue 2

Therapist: *OK, now what I'd like to do is set up the plan for this session. First, I think it's important for us to discuss why it is that organization skills are so important for people with ADHD. After that, I'd like to move on to specifically describing two techniques that will help you to more organized: a calendar system, and a task list system. This discussion will prepare you to choose these and to begin working with them on your own before our next meeting. How does this sound to you?*

Client: *That sounds good to me.*

Discuss why Organizational Skills are so Important for People with ADHD

At this time, the therapist should introduce the rationale for why OTMP skill building is important for most college students with ADHD. This may draw on material from the Background for Therapists for this module (see above), the manual's introductory chapter, and other knowledge regarding ADHD that the therapist has accumulated in his or her experience. This presentation does not need to be lengthy but should remind clients why these skills are critical to their success, thereby bolstering motivation to fully participate in therapy. One tool that the therapist might utilize in such a discussion is a measure of academically oriented skills that includes OTMP, if available (e.g., Parent Academic Management Scale; Sibley, 2017). A model introduction to these concepts that the therapist can use is shown in Dialogue 3; note that it may be useful to solicit the client(s') thoughts regarding how better OTMP might help them in academics and other aspects of their lives.

Dialogue 3

Therapist: Let's talk about organization. In high school, what were you responsible for managing by yourself in school?

Client: Well, let me think. Sometimes I had to do papers and I had to do research and writing. I had to make sure I knew what my assignments were. I had to make sure I had my backpack every day, and that it had the things in it I needed for school. I had tests that I needed to study for, and needed to know when they were.

Therapist: Okay, so that's a lot of things to keep straight. How was it for you doing these things?

Client: I'm not going to lie, it was hard. I mean, sometimes I got stuff done, but it was really hard for me to keep track of everything and to make sure that I finished things when they were due, especially big projects.

Therapist: So, how did you try to help yourself do this?

Client: Well, I kept lists, but sometimes I lost them. I also would make notes to myself in my notebooks, but I forgot to look at them a lot. Mostly my parents and teachers would remind me of things.

Therapist: So is it fair to say that it was a struggle?

Client: Yes.

Therapist: You are not alone in that. Most high schoolers with ADHD struggle to organize themselves and keep up. Remember how we talked about ADHD being a disorder of executive functioning? People with ADHD develop skills like planning and persistence more slowly than others and may in fact always have some difficulty in these areas. But you made it through high school, and now you're in college. Do you think that it is easier for you to be organized and to keep up with your schoolwork and the other things you need to do, now?

Client: No! Professors ask me to do tons more on my own than I did in high school, and we meet less often. I also have to get myself to class and all of my meetings. And my parents aren't nagging and bugging me about these things, either!

Therapist: So is it fair to say that having some tools to keep you on track would be helpful?

Client: Definitely.

Choosing a Calendar System

The first step to improving OTMP is to choose and start using a calendar system. The calendar can be a paper or electronic one. Each student should choose a calendar system that they believe would be optimal. Some students will report having tried a calendar system in the past and having been unsuccessful. One of the goals of this module is to provide structure for students to use the calendar system regularly until its use becomes habitual and to offer advice regarding the pros and cons of different features. It is likely that students who have tried to use a calendar in the past and have been unsuccessful did not use it regularly enough (i.e., at least daily) or did not use it for a long enough period. Such experiences may set up some understandable resistance from student clients regarding completing this step, as they may have concerns about life being "too scheduled." In such instances, it is crucial that the therapist reflects both empathy for these perspectives but also remains steadfast regarding the use of a calendar system. It is very difficult to effectively organize, manage one's time, or specifically plan without a written record to work from, and that should be the consistent message. This is, as far as OTMP goes, the necessary lifeline.

Calendar systems commonly used by our students and colleagues include paper-and-pencil planners, *Google Calendar*, *Outlook*, and *Apple Calendar*. It is alright, and in fact to be expected, that one size will not fit all here, but one important factor in selection is that it is important to choose a calendar that one can always have available. Most college students have already developed the habit of always having their phone with them, and as such we usually start by encouraging students to identify and use electronic calendars that are smartphone-based. Other salient benefits of this choice include the possibility of online or computer-based back-up for such calendars and a high functional and financial cost of *losing* the device in the first place, which might help motivate less misplacement. However, some students may prefer a paper-and-pencil calendar, and this is generally fine, again if it is in a size and format that the student can commit to always having on them, either in a pocket, a backpack, purse, or other means. See Dialogue 4 for a sample discussion of calendar systems.

Dialogue 4

Therapist: *OK, so probably the number one personal organization tool that successful college students and professionals use is a good calendar system. This serves like an external hard drive or bulletin board, where you keep reminders of where you need to be and what you need to do and when. Once you have entered that information, you no longer need to remember it all the time ... all you need to do is to remember to use your calendar!*

Client: *Yeah, I tried using a calendar that my parents gave me in high school. It didn't work so well.*

Therapist: *Can you tell me more about what happened?*

Client: *Well, I had it on my desk at home, and when I got back from school I was supposed to write assignment and test dates on it, and it was supposed to keep me on track. The problem is that sometimes I would forget to write things, and eventually I just stopped using it and went back to my lists on papers I carried.*

Therapist:	*Ah, I see. So it was inconvenient to use?*
Client:	*I guess that's mostly it. And I didn't see the point. I could keep up with things with my lists.*
Therapist:	*How about now, with what you're doing in college? Do you feel confident that your lists will keep you organized?*
Client:	*Not really. There's a lot more things I need to do, and they're more complicated and bigger than before.*
Therapist:	*If we could find a calendar system that worked for you, say, one that is on your iPhone, do you think you would be willing to give it a try? Wouldn't it be nice to be able to carry that with you, and to be able to look at it during the day and know what you need to do?*
Client:	*I think I would be willing to try that, yes.*

Choosing a Task List System

The second step toward effective OTMP is to choose and start using a task or to-do list system. The task list may be integrated with the calendar system (e.g., list within *Outlook* or *Google Calendar*) or separate from it (e.g., a pad of paper or *Wunderlist*). The calendar is used for keeping track of appointments and managing time. The task list is used for keeping track of assignments and other related tasks that one needs to find time to complete.

Task list systems commonly used by our students and colleagues include paper-and-pencil lists, sticky notes, dry-erase boards, *Wunderlist*, *Google Calendar* list, *Apple Notes*, and *Apple Reminders*. Again, the advantage of electronic lists is that they can be readily accessed. Applications like *Wunderlist* are internet-based and can be accessed from any computer or smartphone. In addition, electronic calendar applications can double as a task list by entering tasks to be completed on the current day or later, depending on the urgency. For instance, one student noted that he schedules tasks as "all day" events in his electronic daily calendar, which tend to be highlighted and easy to see in the schedule and yet do not interfere with hour-to-hour appointment or activity listings. Such "events" (or, in this case, tasks) can also be set to repeat such that they appear every day until completed, when the student can delete future occurrences of the task. For several reasons, largely related to convenience and accessibility, we generally encourage our students who own smartphones to start using the embedded electronic calendar and task list as soon as possible. First, it is easier to make sure that you always have your calendar and task list with you if they are electronic. Second, it is easier to lose, and harder to find, a paper-and-pencil calendar or list than it is to lose a smartphone. Most of us are highly motivated to always keep our smartphone with us (e.g., compare the cost of such a device and a piece of paper) and, if we misplace it, we can call it or track it electronically. Third, our society is generally moving in the direction of widespread adoption of phone-based organizational applications, so students who were less comfortable with electronic calendars and task lists can use the support provided through this treatment program to become more comfortable with these technological tools. See Dialogue 5 for a sample discussion of task list systems.

Dialogue 5

Therapist: We've talked about using a calendar to keep you on track with the "when you need to be doing things" part of life, and a very important additional tool is an effective task list system that will keep you on track with the "what you need to be doing" part of life. A lot of people have informal ways of doing this, that are used only every once in a while, like when they are really busy. However, for people with ADHD, it can be especially important to make this an everyday habit, as both the distractibility and the impulsivity can make it really difficult for them to effectively stay on task and be planful about switching to important activities during "free time."

Client: Yeah, I can relate to that.

Therapist: Well, good. Actually, most people can, but again this may be an especially important practice for you. Let's talk about it a bit. Start with what you're doing now: I think you said you keep lists of things you need to do, right? Tell me more about that.

Client: OK. So, basically, when I think of it and particularly when I am busy, I make a list, like on a sticky note or something, and I keep it with me in my pocket or my backpack.

Therapist: Alright, so how does that work for you?

Client: Well, it's not great. First, these things often get lost. I will take it out and put it on the desk in the library, and forget it. Or wash my jeans, and it's in the pocket. Or just drop it, or it gets scrunched at the bottom of my backpack.

Therapist: I see. So, it sounds like this is not working that well. When you do remember to use and actually have the list, though, would you say it helps?

Client: Oh, definitely. I have a hard time remembering everything I need to do on any given day.

Therapist: Alright. Again, this is not unusual. Let's talk about some different options to make your task list more accessible and also more regular, so that you can begin to track what you need to do more effectively.

Homework and Setting the Next Meeting

The therapist should instruct students to choose a calendar system and a task list system, to begin using them, and to bring these along with syllabi and any other work or personal schedules and plans to the next session (see Dialogue 6). It is vital that the therapist emphasizes this strongly, as progress in the next session depends on it. Students should also bring all their course syllabi for the semester to the next session. Finally, make sure that you specifically note with the client(s) what day, time, and place the next session will be. Also, you may want to ask your client if he or she would like you to send a text message reminder the day before the next appointment. We typically recommend that therapists send reminders in the first few weeks of treatment but then talk to clients about phasing these out as the clients begin to use their calendar and personal reminder systems more consistently.

Dialogue 6

Therapist: Today we've talked mainly about calendar and task list systems, and I think we've made progress. You've learned about how these things can add important structure to your daily life, and potentially better keep you on track to success in college. I'm wondering what you think, at this point. Do you think that choosing and using a regular calendar and task list will help?

Client: I think it could. I know that when I actually do use my lists now it helps.

Therapist: It sounds like you would like to try this out.

Client: Yeah!

Therapist: Great! So what I would like you to do – tonight, if possible – is do some more thinking about what sort of calendar you want to use, and what sort of task list, too. Maybe you can look at some paper options, at a store like Staples or OfficeMax or Walmart, and maybe you can look at some electronic options, like on your phone. Remember to focus on how accessible and user-friendly the options are, for you. Choose a calendar you like, and choose a task list system that will complement it. You can start using these if you like, but next time we will mainly be working on getting your calendar and task list set up as well as we can. Because of this, it's really, really important for you to bring your course syllabi, work schedule, and times of any other regular or scheduled commitments you have for this term. Think you can do this?

Client: Yeah, sure, I got it.

Therapist: Great! Now let's make sure we both know when the next time is that we'll meet. Would it be helpful if I sent you a text message reminder the day before our next meeting?

Client:	*Yes, that would be helpful.*
Therapist:	*Okay. I will do that and I will also remind you to bring your syllabi.*

Reference

Sibley, M.H., Comer, J.S., & Gonzalez, J. (2017). Delivering parent-teen therapy for ADHD through videoconferencing: A preliminary investigation. *Journal of Psychopathology and Behavioral Assessment, 39*(3), 467–485. 10.1007/s10862-017-9598-6

Session 2: Beginning and Continuing to Use a Calendar and Task List System

Corresponds to Module 1.2 in the *Thriving in College* Student Workbook

Session Outline

1 Check in with client
2 Set agenda
3 Review homework: Assess materials that client has brought for today (syllabi, schedules, calendar)
4 Use of calendar and task list: Jumpstarting, Maintaining, and Refining
5 Discuss homework
6 Set time and date for the next meeting

Session Organization

Administration Format

Session 2 should be administered in an individual format. An individual session is recommended so that the therapist can support the student in setting up his or her calendar and task list systems and transferring all pertinent information from his or her course syllabi. However, a small group with therapist co-leaders could also be an effective option, if necessary.

Materials Needed

The therapist should bring a whiteboard, flipchart, or projected document to capture group ideas. It is also strongly recommended that the therapist have a laptop computer or tablet with Wi-Fi or other internet connectivity available for this session (see later). Students should bring their calendar and task list to this session. In addition, they need to bring all of their course syllabi for the semester. It is recommended that the therapist send a text message reminder to the student regarding these materials.

DOI: 10.4324/9781003149590-7

Session Content

Check in with Client

As in Session 1, check-in time is used to solicit brief discussion, or simply to see how things are going and build rapport, and should be brief (< 5 minutes), with the therapist encouraging any additional discussion of this sort to be postponed until after the session content is completed (see Dialogue 1). As review of homework from last session is built into the session later, think of this as small talk that eases both therapist and client into the session. Topics might include inquiry into any meaningful events from the last session, how things are going in classes, and other issues that are indicated for the client(s) in question. We also recommend having your client complete the *Progress Tracker* (see Appendix B), and briefly touching base on any declines or improvements in school functioning.

Dialogue 1

Therapist: *It's good to see you today. How have you been doing?*
Client: *Well, alright I guess.*
Therapist: *Do anything interesting over the weekend?*
Client: *Well, yeah, actually I went to see a Sci-fi movie with a friend. I love that kind of movie, it was really good.*
Therapist: *That does sound fun. It's important to find ways to keep a balance while in school.*
Client: *How was your weekend?*
Therapist: *I had a good weekend too, thanks for asking! So, obviously, I want to talk more about organization and time management today. Let's start by setting the agenda, Okay?*

Set Agenda

Introduce the agenda for this session to the client (see Session Outline). As in Session 1, it may be helpful to have a visual aid to refer to, such as a flip chart or projected PowerPoint slide or printed handout, and it might also be helpful to remind clients to take notes. The therapist-client interaction modeled in Session 1 (see earlier) can be adapted slightly for this and all subsequent sessions; remember that this activity should be quite brief (< 2 minutes).

Review Homework

Clients were asked in Session 1 to choose a calendar and a task list system that they will begin using, and to bring documents to this session that are necessary to implement these things (e.g., syllabi). During this part of the session, which again should be brief (~5 minutes), the therapist should directly check with the client if these things have been accomplished (see Dialogue 2). Many clients will have followed the homework instructions, but others will not have, and the therapist will need to adjust accordingly, as follows.

- *If the student arrives for the session without having chosen a calendar and task list system,* the session should be spent helping the student make these decisions and, if necessary, an extra session should be scheduled for transferring dates from their course syllabi.
- *If the student arrives for the session without the calendar and task list system that he or she chose,* then two responses are possible. First, in the case that the student has chosen electronic (e.g., smart-phone-based) options, it may be possible for the therapist to use a laptop or tablet to "pull up" the calendar and task list via an online account. Second, in the case that the student has chosen a paper-based calendar and/or task list system, it is advisable to reschedule this appointment, as these are necessary to complete the activities herein.
- *If a student arrives without his or her course syllabi,* again, it may be possible for the therapist to access this online through a university or college system (e.g., Blackboard, Canvas). If even one or two syllabi can be accessed in this way the therapist can effectively coach the client (see Dialogue 2). If this is not possible, the session should be rescheduled, and the client should be reminded that these materials are vital to achieving the goals of the session.

Dialogue 2

Therapist:	*The main thing that we'll be focusing on today is using your calendar and task list. First, I want to make sure we're ready for that: Do you have your calendar, task list, and other materials with you?*
Client:	*Uh, well, yeah, I am using the Apple Calendar and Reminders apps that are on my phone, and I have that. What other materials were there?*
Therapist:	*We talked about bringing your syllabi and your work schedule with you today so that we could make sure those things were reflected accurately in your new system.*
Client:	*Oh. Whoops. I forgot about those.*
Therapist:	*Hmm* (therapist smiles encouragingly at client) *this seems like something that could have been helped with a calendar or a task list, eh?*
Client:	*Ha. Yeah.*
Therapist:	*Well, tell you what … do any of your professors have an online course website with a syllabus that we could look at today, so we could continue?*

> *Client:*   *Totally! All of them! Do you want me to pull it up on my phone?*
> *Therapist:* *Yes, if that's convenient, or we could use my laptop. Either way, let's do that now.*

Note that in any of these cases, problem-solving regarding a student's forgetfulness is encouraged. In fact, this can be an opportunity for the therapist to reinforce that the successful implementation of these organizational tools is important and will lead to better success.

It is also possible that clients will not only have chosen their calendar and task list, but also will have begun, on their own, to use them. The *Jumpstarting Calendar and Task List System* section can proceed basically as written in this instance, although the therapist should make sure to reinforce the client's initial efforts with verbal praise and engage in a discussion about how the client finds these systems to work so far. This instance will also allow more focus on refining and troubleshooting during the session (see *Refining the Use of Calendar and Task List,* below).

Jumpstarting Calendar and Task List System

Once students have chosen a calendar and task list system, the next step is to add all classes and appointments to their calendars. Some students will resist the idea of adding regularly scheduled commitments to their calendar. They might argue that they do not tend to forget to go to their classes once they have memorized their schedules (although they may admit to choosing not to go). In such cases, it may be helpful for the therapist to employ aspects of motivational interviewing or similar approaches to bolster cooperation and follow-through. For instance, pros and cons for complete adoption of the calendar system can be reviewed, as can the short- and potential long-term benefits, to motivate the reluctant. For some students, entering all class meeting times and regular appointments into the calendar is helpful for making sure they do not forget to go to class. However, it is more important for being able to visually assess how much time a student has available to complete other things on his or her task list before, after, or in-between classes or regularly scheduled appointment (e.g., a part-time job) and, thus, learn to manage time (see Dialogue 3). Once students have entered all their class meeting times and regularly scheduled commitments into their calendars, students are asked to transfer all assignments, exam dates, and due dates from their course syllabi to their calendars and task lists. Note that it is also important to cue students to include planned personal or extracurricular events on their calendars, as well, so that these can be accurately figured into planning and time management. This all can be a very overwhelming task the first time it is undertaken. Therefore, we ask students to bring their calendars, task lists and syllabi to this second session for as much hands-on assistance as is needed. Once students have gone through this process with all their syllabi for one or two semesters, they are usually less overwhelmed by this task, and they appreciate its usefulness to a much greater degree.

Dialogue 3

Therapist: *Now we've got all your syllabi and your work and extracurricular schedules here, and it's time to get down to putting all the regular meetings and also assignment, test, and personal dates in your calendar. Where would you like to start?*

Client: *I guess let's start with test and paper due dates.* (Client puts these from all syllabi in calendar with support from Therapist.)

Therapist: *OK, that's a great start! Now, one thing that you'll probably want to do is to put reminders and planned times for preparing for these tests in your calendar, too, but you will first need to know exactly **when** those blocks of time will be available. To get closer to that, let's now put in all of your scheduled classes, work, and other commitments.*

Client: *Really? That's a lot to do. I don't know if I need that, either. I mean, I remember when my classes are and stuff.*

Therapist: *Well that's good. In fact, that may put you at an advantage compared to some other people who have ADHD. But here's the thing: We know that people with ADHD can sometimes have a hard time accurately anticipating how much time it takes to get things done, and they can also simply lose track of time. Does that ever happen for you?*

Client: *Well, yeah, it does.*

Therapist: *By putting **all** your scheduled appointments and classes and work in your calendar, it will begin to help you notice and plan the use of your time better, and help you to not be caught expecting to have more time for something than you really do. It does seem like a lot of work, I know, but it gets easier and the payoff is less stress, better readiness for tests and other assignments, and fewer missed opportunities. Does this make sense? Are you willing to try it?*

Client: *Sure, it does make sense to me, now. I'm willing to try.* (Client completes calendar with support from Therapist.)

Maintaining Use of a Calendar and Task List System

The final step for using this organizational system is one that will be ongoing. Specifically, the student should be checking and updating their calendar and task list regularly. We typically suggest that this be done three times per day, and that it is helpful to yoke it to a daily activity (e.g., while drinking coffee in the morning and afternoon, and then again while brushing teeth at night). Clients should be encouraged to develop the habit of doing this. For example, a student might check his or her calendar and task list at night before going to bed to get an overview of what the next day will look like, and again in the morning before leaving the house. It does not matter when students check their calendars and task lists, as long as they get in the habit of referencing them several times a day.

Students should also become accustomed to updating their calendars immediately when they schedule a new appointment, receive a new assignment, or think of something that needs to be completed. If a student reports at subsequent sessions that he or she is not checking and updating their calendar or task list on at least a daily basis, then the system is not working, and the therapist will need to problem-solve with the student. It may be that the student needs to choose a different calendar or task list system or that the student needs to try alternative strategies for remembering to check their calendar or task list regularly (e.g., setting a reminder on smartphone). If none of these are the case, then it might be necessary to use some motivational interviewing techniques to help the client appreciate the advantages of checking the calendar regularly.

Refining the Use of Calendar and Task List

Often our clients will come in and tell us that things are already going well with their calendar and task list. The clinician might be tempted to accept this and move on to the next skill. It is our recommendation that the therapist and client look at the calendar and task list together to determine if the client is using these tools optimally. See Dialogue 4 for a sample discussion between the therapist and client.

Dialogue 4

Therapist: *How did it go with using your new calendar and task list systems this week?*

Client: *It went pretty well. I am using the google calendar with my gmail account and Trello for my task list.*

Therapist: *Would you mind pulling up your calendar on this computer so that we take a look?*

Client: *Sure.*

Client opens calendar and therapist can see that only a few events are entered into the calendar (e.g., a doctor's appointment, an advising appointment) but no classes or assignments.

Therapist: *Okay. I see that you have some appointments in your calendar which is a good start. A lot of students find it helpful to also enter their classes into the calendar.*

Client:	*That doesn't seem necessary to me because I know when my classes are and they follow the same schedule every week and I don't usually forget to go to class.*
Therapist:	*I understand that forgetting to go to class is not a problem for you. Can you think of any advantages of adding your classes to the calendar.*
Client:	*Not really.*
Therapist:	*Some students have told us that they find it really helpful to be able to see how many hours in the day are left for studying and doing things on their task list.*
Client:	*I guess that might be helpful.*
Therapist:	*If you are willing to give it a try, we could go ahead and enter your classes into the calendar now and then start discussing when you might have time to do some of the things on your task list this week?*
Client:	*Okay. That sounds good.*

The following additional steps may be implemented with clients to enhance the usefulness of the calendar system as deemed appropriate for individual clients. Therapists should introduce each of these additional strategies and provide examples.

Use a Calendar to Keep Track of How Much Time Is Spent on Tasks

Many of us have had the experience of tasks taking longer than we planned. In addition, many of us have thought that there are not enough hours in the day to complete all the things that we need to do. Individuals with ADHD have more difficulty in estimating how much time has passed or how long it will take to finish something. Because unrealistic task-time estimates can sabotage students' effort to improve OTMP and related academic performance (e.g., motivation sags after repeated late- or all-nighters to finish tasks where required effort was poorly judged), it may be most helpful to incorporate this kind of exercise early in the OTMP intervention in order to heighten the realism of early planning efforts. One exercise that is often helpful for improving time estimation is to keep a log of how one's time is spent over the course of a few days. If a person learns that making dinner, eating dinner and doing the dishes consistently takes 45 minutes, then she will know how much time to accurately allocate for that activity in the future.

Schedule Homework and Breaks on Calendar

Another option is to use the calendar not only for keeping track of appointments and classes but also for planning out how one will spend one's time in the days ahead and for noting how time was spent in the current day. Aspects of urgent and important tasks from the task list (see prioritization, introduced below) should be scheduled for completion in the coming few days. In our experience, tasks are much more likely to be completed and not to fall through the cracks if we *specifically* plan out when we will work on them (see Dialogue 5).

Dialogue 5

Therapist: *It can be helpful to use your calendar to keep track of how you spent your time each day. Even if you don't choose to use this as a regular strategy, it can be helpful to keep track of how you spent your time for a few days to get a better sense of where the time is going and how long things take. Look at this example:*

	Monday	Tuesday	Wednesday
8am	*Wake-up & get ready*	*Wake-up & get ready*	*Wake-up & get ready*
9am	**Chemistry class**	*Chemistry homework*	**Chemistry class**
10am	**Psychology class**	*Chemistry homework*	**Psychology class**
11am	**Statistics class**	*Chemistry homework*	**Statistics class**
12pm	*Lunch*	*Lunch*	*Lunch*
1pm	**Study group**	**Chemistry lab**	*Chemistry homework*
2pm	**Study group**	**Chemistry lab**	*Chemistry homework*
3pm	**Advising appointment**	**Chemistry lab**	*Chemistry homework*
4pm	*Exercise*	*Exercise*	*Exercise*
5pm	*Shower*	*Shower*	*Shower*
6pm	*Dinner*	*Dinner*	*Dinner*
7pm	**Club meeting**	**Statistics tutor**	*Clean bathroom*
8pm	*Laundry*	*Psychology homework*	*Statistics homework*
9pm	*Laundry*	*Psychology homework*	*Statistics homework*
10pm	*Laundry*	*Psychology homework*	*Statistics homework*

Therapist: *In this example schedule, the items that are in bold are actual classes or appointments whereas the items that are in italicized text are things from the student's task list. This allows the student to visualize when things will get done. Do you think this might work for you?*

Client: *I can't imagine being that structured. I don't usually plan ahead like that. I prefer to be spontaneous.*

Therapist: *I understand that it might sound a bit inflexible to you. Keep in mind that it is a plan that you can alter as needed. Students have told us that this has really helped them to increase their productivity.*

Client: *I guess I would be willing to give it a try for a few days.*

Therapist: *Let's go ahead and plan out the rest of your day today and tomorrow in this way and then you can give it a try and let me know how it worked the next time I see you.*

The therapist should help the client plan out the next day or two in the session. It is our experience that clients are much less likely to give this time management exercise a try if it is assigned as homework rather than something that happens in session with therapist support. The therapist and client will plan out 1 or 2 days together and then it can be recommended that the client plan out the rest of the week on their own.

Reschedule Unfinished, Scheduled Tasks for Tomorrow

If two hours were allocated today for finishing an English paper and it was not completed (either in that allotted amount of time or due to task avoidance), the student should schedule some time in the next day or two to finish it. This process will also help the client to gain a better sense of how long it will take to complete similar tasks and assignments.

Make Better Use of Time Cracks in One's Day

Solanto (2010) coined the term "time cracks" to describe short spans that one may be tempted to waste on meaningless activity (e.g., surfing the Web, watching Netflix) that otherwise, if used wisely, could facilitate task completion. Coaching students to notice such brief opportunities during their day and to search their task lists for items that can be quickly resolved can help to maintain a sense of accomplishment throughout the day and instill adaptive task orientation.

Discuss Homework and Set the Next Meeting

Students should check and update their calendars and task lists at least twice a day (but, as noted above, three is recommended) and make note of any difficulties encountered. It is also encouraged that each student try some of the additional calendar-use strategies prior to the next session, as a means of broadening skill development. Finally, make sure that you specifically note with the client(s) what day, time, and place the next session will be, and that calendars and task lists should be brought to the next meeting for review and troubleshooting (as needed).

Reference

Solanto, M.V., Marks, D.J., Wasserstein, J., Mitchell, K., Abikoff, H., Alvir, J.M., & Kofman, M.D. (2010). Efficacy of meta-cognitive therapy for adult ADHD. *The American Journal of Psychiatry, 167*(8), 958–968. 10.1176/appi.ajp.2009.09081123

Session 3: Task Prioritization and Sustaining Behavior through Rewards and Accountability

Corresponds to Modules 1.3 and 1.4 in the
Thriving in College Student Workbook

Session Outline

1 Check in with client
2 Set agenda
3 Review homework: Examine and discuss use of calendar, task list, strategies
4 Teaching effective task prioritization
5 Rewards for successful task completion
6 Establishing accountability: Self and friends
7 Discuss homework/follow-up
8 (As needed) Set time and date for next meeting

Session Organization

Administration Format

Session 3 can be administered in a group or individual format. A group session is optimal, but an individual session is acceptable if a group session is not indicated (e.g., therapist has just one or two appropriate clients) or practical.

Materials Needed

The therapist should bring a whiteboard, flipchart, or projected document to capture group ideas regarding prioritization (and markers, if appropriate) and prioritization grid handout or display. Students should bring their task lists and calendars.

Session Content

Check-in with Client

As in previous sessions, check-in time is used to solicit brief discussion, or simply to see how things are going and further build rapport, and should be brief (< 5 minutes), encouraging any additional discussion of this sort to be postponed until after the session content is completed. Remember, this time is not specifically

DOI: 10.4324/9781003149590-8

for review of homework, which comes later. Clinicians could inquire here about any meaningful events since the last session, how things are going in classes, and other topics that are indicated given the clients' history and the session context (i.e., individual or group). The check-in dialogue from Session 2 (see earlier) could be adapted with only minimal alteration for this session. We also recommend having your client complete the *Progress Tracker* (see Appendix B), and briefly touching base on any declines or improvements in school functioning.

Setting Agenda

Introduce the agenda for this session to the client (see earlier). As in previous sessions, it may be helpful to have a visual aid for this. The therapist is encouraged to again remind the client(s) to take notes, and to keep this brief (< 2 minutes).

Review Homework.

Clients were asked in Session 2 to begin using the calendar and a task list system that they chose, to consider adapting one or more of the supplemental strategies for time management that were introduced, and to bring their calendar and task list today. During this part of the session, which again should be brief (~5 minutes), the therapist should directly check with the client(s) if these things have been accomplished (see Dialogue 1). Depending on how well each client has been able to complete these tasks, the therapist may need to adjust accordingly, as follows.

1 *If the client does not arrive with his or her calendar* (and it is not electronically accessible), instead of a visual check-in, discuss progress in utilizing this tool. In this case, inquire as to the degree of detail the client is using in the calendar. Are all regular classes entered? Work hours? Extracurricular and social engagements? Are assignments broken down and components noted in the calendar, with time allotted for completion? Are holidays and deadlines noted? Emphasize that the calendar is only effective as a planning and time management tool if it captures all these various aspects of daily life. (If the client *does* have the calendar accessible, visual examination and conversation should be around these principles, as well.)

2 *If the client does not arrive with his or her task list* (and this is not electronically accessible), then the session may proceed but the therapist will have to ask the client to recall/generate tasks for use in discussing task prioritization (see later). Whether the client has access to the task list or not, the therapist should ask about the frequency with which the client is referring to the list and the perceived utility of its use. If the client is not combining the use of calendar and task list (i.e., not noting times assigned or deadlines for tasks to be completed), the therapist should coach the client on this further and employ motivational techniques to bolster the likelihood of adopting this behavior.

3   *If the client reports that he or she has not tried any of the additional strategies* for calendar use that were presented in Session 2 (i.e., using it to track time spent on tasks, scheduling homework and breaks, rescheduling unfinished tasks, making use of "time cracks"), then briefly remind the client of these and inquire as to why the client chose to omit this step. Encourage the client to think further about these strategies and to adopt them to maximize the effectiveness of their time management behavior, focusing on building client motivation.

Dialogue 1

Therapist: *You were asked to do a lot since last session, and I want to review how that went. First, you were asked to start using the iPhone calendar and task list you chose last time, to put those things into practice. Second, you were asked to try some of the additional strategies for calendar and task list use that I described last session. Third, you were asked to bring your calendar and task list back today so we could talk more about those. How did all of this go?*

Client: *Pretty good, I think. I have put my classes and work times into my calendar, and I created a task list and have been checking things off and adding new tasks as I've needed to. I think I've been using some of the strategies, too … the thing I remember and have been trying is making use of my time cracks.*

Therapist: *Great! It sounds like you are making some changes that could be helping … what do you think, do these help?*

Client: *I think so, yes. I feel a little less anxious with everything written down like this. I didn't miss a single class last week, and usually I do.*

Therapist: *Well, if you keep it up, hopefully missing class will be a thing of the past. How often are you looking at your calendar and your task list?*

Client: *I look at my calendar in the morning and in the evening when I get home and settled to do schoolwork in the evening. I sometimes look at it at other times during the day too, if I'm not sure about what I have to do. I look at my task list at those times too, and then also when I have free time.*

Therapist: *Sounds like you are starting to make this a habit, and I think you are really going to benefit from it. I'm wondering whether you have put deadlines for assignments and also components of larger tasks, like studying for tests or researching topics for a term paper, into your calendar, too?*

Client: *I've done some of that. Would you like to see?*

Therapist: *Yes, that would be great.*

Therapist reviews the client's calendar, making reinforcing comments as warranted and also providing guidance on fine tuning, as needed.

Teaching Effective Task Prioritization

Once a task list is established, it can still be difficult to decide what to do first or when to start a task in order to complete it by the due date. One strategy for determining the order in which tasks should be completed is to assign priority ratings (e.g., A for things that should be completed as soon as possible, B for things that are less urgent, and C for things that can wait even longer). Another strategy is to evaluate each item on the task list in terms of urgency and importance. It is informative to work through a list of tasks as a group and see if group members (or individual clients) agree regarding which things are urgent and important. Inevitably, it will become clear that there are different judgments about which things are urgent and important. For example, some students may argue that dishes need to be washed immediately so that they do not stack up and other students may purport that doing dishes is not urgent or important. Such individual differences are to be expected, and yet the discussions surrounding such decisions can particularly help the client with ADHD to develop a balanced understanding of "urgency" and "importance." The grids shown in Box 1 can be used to demonstrate how task list items might be categorized using relative urgency and importance, and also as a worksheet to complete with clients in session utilizing their own to-do tasks (blank copy also included in Appendix A).

Box 1 In-session task prioritization worksheet

Urgent and important: • Writing English paper due tomorrow • Finishing chemistry assignment due Monday	Not urgent but important • Writing Sociology paper due in four weeks • Updating resume for summer jobs
Urgent but not important: • Washing dishes • Grocery shopping for the week	Not urgent and not important: • Buying a new video game • Selling basketball ticket that I cannot use
Urgent and important:	Not urgent but important:
Urgent but not important:	Not urgent and not important:

Adapted from Covey (1989).

Based on this grid, it is easy to realize that the tasks that are *urgent and important* (e.g., ones that relate to tests or academic assignments with deadlines in the next few days) should probably be completed first. The tasks that are *important but not urgent* are ones that could wait a few days (e.g., starting to organize and research a paper due in three weeks). However, these might also be good tasks to set aside some time in the next few days to get started on, even though their completion is not especially urgent. The tasks that are *urgent but not important* are often ones related to daily living and might be good options for a study break (e.g., going to the grocery store to restock for the coming week). Students might consider eliminating the tasks that are *not urgent and not important* from their lists altogether. For example, buying a new video game might not need to be on someone's list because, if you forget, there are not dire consequences, and it is likely that a student would be motivated to remember. Alternatively, selling an extra basketball ticket could be considered important if the student really needed the money. However, since in the aforementioned example the student in question categorized this item as not urgent and not important it is likely that they do not really badly need the money. Also, this student will probably remember to offer up their ticket if they hear other students discussing wanting to go to the basketball game.

A possible pitfall in task prioritization is that if one has lots of A's *that truly are urgent and important* and also require significant effort, the task list itself can be perceived as aversive and overwhelming. Therapists may need to be flexible and help their clients to think similarly, encouraging sporadic prioritization of an "easy" B or C task to maintain motivation and energy to tackle the task list. While this will be covered in detail in the next session, it may also be helpful to mention to overwhelmed clients the principle of breaking larger tasks down to create some steps that are *urgent and important* and others that are *important but not urgent.* Simply telling the client about this and that it will be something to work on in the future can help reduce overwhelmed feelings and get them to think about this and maybe try it a little on their own before the next session.

Rewards for Successful Task Completion

Another useful strategy is to schedule breaks or rewards for oneself during the day. Many of our students have reported spending too much time playing video games or watching Netflix or using Facebook when they should be studying. One way to address this problem is for students to set goals and then reward oneself with an enjoyable activity after having completed the goal. For example, a student could make an agreement with herself that she will watch one 20-minute episode of *Friends* on Netflix for every hour of studying or homework she completes. This strategy has been referred to as the *when-then rule* or the *Premack Principle*. Here are some additional examples:

1 **When** I finish my chemistry homework, **then** I will watch an episode of *The Big Bang Theory*.
2 **When** I have chosen a topic for my term paper, **then** I will play *Call of Duty* for 30 minutes.
3 **When** I finish the first page of my English paper, **then** I will go for a run.
4 **When** I finish washing the breakfast dishes, **then** I will eat lunch.
5 **When** I finish reading this chapter, **then** I will do my grocery shopping.

It is important to note that each student must determine which rewards will be personally motivating. It may be that grocery shopping does not sound that exciting but, if it is less aversive for you than reading your textbook, this agreement with yourself may be successful. It is also important that therapists confer basic principles regarding the *appropriateness* of different rewards for various accomplishments. For example, choosing a term paper topic—not the most difficult or time-consuming task—should probably not call for a large and potentially disruptive reward (e.g., going out of town to attend a concert, or even watching a feature-length movie), whereas finishing one's last take-home exam for the term certainly could.

Establishing Accountability: Hold Yourself Accountable

Making "deals" with yourself regarding fun or at least, less aversive activities, is one strategy for helping increase motivation. It is also useful to discuss other strategies for holding oneself accountable or increasing the likelihood that you will remember to follow through with a plan. Some additional strategies include: (a) establishing routines and rituals, (b) strategic scheduling, (c) using "implementation intentions," and (d) being "strict" with yourself. We will discuss each of these four strategies in more detail.

First, creating new routines and rituals can be an effective means of increasing motivation and decreasing procrastination. For example, a student who has difficulty keeping up with laundry and tends to avoid this chore until she has no clean clothes to wear might decide to establish a routine regarding laundry. The routine could include pairing an aversive chore with a rewarding activity such as doing laundry on Sunday evenings, after several hours of studying, and watching Netflix or playing video games in between folding and transferring laundry. By pairing the laundry with screen time, the student may stop procrastinating on doing laundry. In addition, the combination of laundry and screen time might also become a reward for productive studying on Sunday afternoons.

Second, strategic scheduling can be used to optimize productivity. For example, a student with ADHD may have difficulty being productive with schoolwork in the evenings when his medication has worn off, and he may *also* be struggling with his calculus course, which is not uncommon for college students regardless of ADHD status. If he scheduled a math tutor on Mondays at 7pm, this might provide the necessary structure to help him be productive at this time of day. Another option would be to schedule a study group for this time rather than scheduling the study group at 2pm when the student is more likely to be productive independently.

Third, there is some evidence that implementation intentions can be a helpful strategy for remembering to do something at a future time or increasing the likelihood that you will follow through. The term "implementation intention" was introduced by Gollwitzer (1999) and it is a strategy for self-regulation. Implementation intentions are plans that a person makes to complete a task in the future when cued by an event or stimulus in the environment. Part of the strategy for increasing the likelihood that the implementation intention will work is to imagine oneself doing the task. Here are some examples of implementation intentions:

1 When my psychology class is over, I will go to the library and study. (Imagine yourself walking from the psychology building to the library rather than walking to your dorm as usual.)
2 When I get home and go to the refrigerator for a snack (which I always do), I will sit down at the kitchen table and begin reading for my political science class. (Imagine yourself going to refrigerator, obtaining snack, sitting down at table, pulling out textbook and beginning to read.)
3 I have been having trouble remembering to call student health to schedule an appointment to see my prescribing physician, and I am almost out of my stimulant medication. I keep remembering in the evening when student health is closed. When I go home for lunch, I will call the student health service to schedule an appointment. (Imagine yourself going home for lunch, putting food in the microwave and calling student health while you are waiting for food to warm-up.)

Finally, students may need to learn to be "stricter" with themselves. If you make a deal with yourself that you will not watch your favorite television show until you have finished your sociology paper and you do not follow-through, then this type of accountability strategy will be less likely to work in the future. Students should be advised to make realistic goals when they strike deals with themselves. It is not recommended to commit to writing an entire paper in one sitting and then depriving yourself of your television show if you do not finish. However, if you set a realistic goal, it is not wise to get into the habit of not holding yourself to it. For example, if you commit to writing the introductory paragraph of your paper before watching your show and you do not get it done, it would be prudent to skip your show until tomorrow night. This might increase your motivation to make sure you finish that first paragraph tomorrow. This might be a good time to remind students that one of the disadvantages of being an adult is that you have to be the one to hold yourself accountable because, ultimately, your success is up to you.

Establishing Accountability: Have Your Friends Hold You Accountable

Some students will have more difficulty employing self-discipline to hold themselves to these types of self-agreements. There are several additional strategies that other students have found helpful. First, a student might want to employ a friend in one or both parts of this agreement. For example, a student could tell his roommate that he really wants to get caught up on the dishes and propose that they both do the dishes together before allowing themselves to make lunch. Alternatively, a student could ask a friend if she would be willing to go for a run or go to the gym together after the student finishes the first page of her English paper. Sometimes, the act of making such a statement to another person is enough to motivate a person to hold herself accountable. Another example would be to make plans with a friend and reserve a study room together at the library to increase the likelihood that you will go to the library in the evening.

Discuss Homework and Set the Next Meeting

The therapist should instruct and encourage the client to continue to check and update their calendar and task list on at least a daily basis and make note of any difficulties encountered. Students should also complete the "urgency and importance grid" using the items from their own task lists and bring it to the next session (see Appendix A for handout). Students should also set up some reward contingencies to try and help sustain and build motivation for difficult tasks. Employ a motivational interviewing style during this discussion, as illustrated in previous sessions' homework-setting discussions. Finally, make sure that you specifically note with the client(s) what day, time, and place the next session will be.

Reference

Gollwitzer, P.M. (1999). Implementation intentions: Strong effects of simple plans. *American Psychologist, 54*(7), 493–503. 10.1037/0003-066X.54.7.493

Session 4: Managing Procrastination

Corresponds to Module 1.5 in the *Thriving in College* Student Workbook

Session Outline

1 Check in with client(s)
2 Set agenda
3 Review homework: Prioritization and rewards
4 Introduce procrastination
5 Breaking tasks down into smaller steps
6 Challenging thoughts and emotions
7 Changing behavioral routines
8 Discuss homework and follow-up

Session Organization

Administration Format

Session 4 can be administered in a group or individual format. A group session is optimal, but an individual session is also acceptable.

Materials Needed

The therapist should bring a whiteboard, flipchart, or projected document to capture group ideas regarding breaking tasks into steps. Students should bring their task lists.

Session Content

Check-in with Client(s)

As in previous sessions, check-in time is used to solicit brief discussion, or simply to see how things are going and further build rapport, and should be brief (< 5 minutes), encouraging for any additional discussion of this sort to be postponed until after the session content is completed. Remember, this time is not specifically for review of homework, which comes later. Clinicians could inquire here about any meaningful events since the last session, how things are going in

DOI: 10.4324/9781003149590-9

classes, and other topics that are indicated given the clients' history and the session context (i.e., individual or group). The check-in dialogue from Session 2 (see earlier) could be adapted with only minimal alteration for this session. We also recommend having your client complete the *Progress Tracker* (see Appendix B), and briefly touching base on any declines or improvements in school functioning.

Setting Agenda

Introduce the agenda for this session to the client (see earlier). As in previous sessions, it may be helpful to have a visual aid for this. The therapist is encouraged to again remind the client(s) to take notes, and to keep this brief (< 2 minutes).

Review Homework

Clients were asked in Session 3 to continue using the calendar and a task list system that they chose, to *start* using task prioritization and reward contingencies, and to bring their associated materials today. During this part of the session, which again should be brief (aim for ~5 minutes), the therapist should directly check whether these things have been accomplished and focus most on troubleshooting and motivating task prioritization and the use of contingencies. Depending on how well the client has been able to complete these tasks, the therapist may need to spend some additional time answering questions about and/or troubleshooting the implementation of these novel strategies. Therapists should also take care to specifically ensure that the client is continuing to *actively* employ his or her calendar and running task list.

Introducing Procrastination

One issue that often arises with task lists, and completing tasks in general, is procrastination. One indicator that clients can use to detect when they are procrastinating is avoidance of the tasks on their list. First, you should discuss with clients the consequences of procrastination which might include increased stress, interference with other things that they were planning to do, a result that is not as good as it could have been, and missing out on social activities, sleep and exercise. It could also result in a product that is simply "acceptable," which might actually increase the likelihood of procrastinating again in the future.

There are several strategies for increasing motivation and decreasing procrastination. First, it may be helpful to break tasks down into smaller steps. Second, students may need to challenge their negative thoughts about the task and how difficult it will be to get started or complete. Third, it may be necessary to change one or more behavioral routines that are preventing the student from getting started or completing the task. In this session, you will discuss each of these three strategies with clients in more detail. The therapist may want to start by helping the client assess whether he or she is having difficulty with motivation and/or procrastination (see Dialogue 1 for an example discussion).

Dialogue 1

Therapist: How have things been going this week in terms of accomplishing tasks on your list?

Client: It's going pretty well.

Therapist: Are there any items on your list that you feel like you have been avoiding?

Client: Yes, there are a couple. One of them is straightening up or organizing my desk and another is writing a term paper for my philosophy class.

Therapist: Do you feel like you have been procrastinating on these items or that you really haven't had the time to get started?

Client: I think I have been procrastinating. Both of these things seem really unpleasant to me. I am overwhelmed by the idea of cleaning my desk because it is such a mess and I don't know where to start with the term paper.

Therapist: What happens when you procrastinate? What are the consequences?

Client: I feel more stressed. Sometimes I think I need to be a little more stressed in order to make myself get started but other times I get so stressed that I feel almost paralyzed. Sometimes I wait until the very last minute to get started and then I have to pull an all-nighter to get it done.

Therapist: Does that work out okay for you in the end?

Client: Not really. I often end up missing out on things that I was planning to do with my roommates and I feel really unproductive for a few days afterwards until I get caught up on my sleep.

Therapist: That doesn't sound like a great outcome, but it might be okay if you end up being satisfied with the paper that you submitted.

Client: I am usually not happy with the paper because I know it's not my best work. I think I would do better if I started the paper earlier and was able to review a couple of drafts before turning it in, but I can't figure out how to make myself get started earlier.

Breaking Tasks Down into Smaller Steps

Therapists and clients should examine items on the list that the client is avoiding. One reason for procrastination might be that the task is too large and overwhelming and needs to be broken down into smaller steps. As a rule of thumb, we tell students, **"If you don't know where to start, then the task is too big."** A college student with ADHD may procrastinate and otherwise avoid writing a five-page term paper if that is perceived as a practically insurmountable task. However, completing this same paper could be broken down into the following steps: (a) choose a topic; (b) conduct literature search; (c) read articles; (d) create an outline; (e) write first page; (f) write second page; (g) write third page; (h) write fourth page; (i) write fifth page; (j) revise first draft; (k) revise second draft; (l) proofread final draft; (m) submit paper to professor. Once these steps have been established, each can be added separately to the student's list of things to do. It is much less likely that he will procrastinate if he sits down to *choose a topic for term paper* than to *write 5-page term paper*. Breaking tasks down into smaller steps can also help us figure out how to allocate our time in order to finish the task by the due date. If a student determines that there are 12 steps involved in writing this term paper and it is due in 14 days, she might set a goal for completing one step a day with two days allowed for breaks from working on it. It is recommended that the therapist and client work through the process of breaking down a couple of tasks into smaller steps so that clients can experience how this process works and also share their experiences in trying to use this strategy with other group members if this session is being administered in a group format. The therapist should solicit examples from students of tasks on their lists that they are having trouble completing and then choose one to work through as a group (see Dialogue 2).

Dialogue 2

Therapist: *You mentioned that you have been having difficulty with organizing your desk.*

Client: *Yes, it is a mess. I have piled lots of stuff on it so I can't work there.*

Therapist: *Okay, let's try using the strategy that we just discussed about breaking tasks down into smaller steps. What are some possible steps that you could take toward getting your desk cleaned?*

Client: *I don't know. I think it would take a couple of hours to do it and I never feel like I have that much time.*

Therapist: *One thing that has worked for others is to get a couple of bags or boxes and take everything off of the desk and put things into boxes or bags. Then you could take care of the things in one of the bags each day and you could start using your desk again right away. Does that sound like it might work for you?*

Client: *Maybe. I like the idea of being able to use my desk again but I'd be a little worried that the bags would sit around for the rest of the semester.*

Therapist: *Yes, I can understand how you might be concerned about that, and it could happen, but it would probably be less likely to happen if you kept the remaining steps on your task list. Let's make a list of the possible steps involved in cleaning your desk and then you can see what you think.*

> *Client:*   Okay. First, I will take everything off of my desk and sort it into bags. I will have one bag for: (1) things that need to go back on my desk; (2) clothes or things that need to be put away in other parts of my apartment; and one for (3) things to be thrown away or recycled.
>
> *Therapist:*   That sounds great. Then you would have four items to enter on your task list including clearing off the desk one day and sorting through each of the bags on the following three days. Do you think that might work for you?
>
> *Client:*   Yes, I will give it a try this week.

Challenging Thoughts and Emotions

Individuals with ADHD are particularly susceptible to maladaptive thinking. Many individuals with ADHD have a clinically significant comorbid depression or anxiety diagnosis; however, even those who do not are more likely to engage in dysfunctional thinking regarding their own ability to accomplish necessary tasks (Knouse & Mitchell, 2015; Strohmeier et al., 2016). Ramsay and Rostain (2016) have argued that many adults with ADHD have problems following through on their behavioral intentions. Further, Knouse and Mitchell (2015) suggest that adults with ADHD can sometimes be *overly* optimistic about their abilities (including ability to complete schoolwork), which presents its own challenges to successful task completion. Thus, establishing a calendar and task list system becomes a necessary but insufficient step in learning to successfully complete one's academic, professional, and/or personal responsibilities. Cognitive behavioral therapy can be used to help students challenge their maladaptive thinking about their ability to complete tasks on their list. For example, if a student has tried using a calendar system in the past but has been unsuccessful, he might believe that he will fail again. Alternatively, if a student has broken her term paper down into 12 steps but still believes that she is not capable of completing one step each day, then she is unlikely to be successful in this endeavor. It is not unusual for clients with ADHD to have experienced multiple failures in their attempts to become organized and productive and that this has impacted their self-efficacy in this regard. For this reason, we recommend that therapists discuss students' confidence in their ability to follow through with their goals, appointments and tasks and help them either challenge negative or maladaptive thoughts or develop more realistic thinking regarding the difficulty of their school and other work as needed in this session.

Changing Behavioral Routines

Another aspect to difficulties with implementation of intentions may involve becoming "stuck" in maladaptive behavioral routines or scripts (Ramsay, 2016).

Students might need to evaluate how their habits or routines are interfering with following through on a plan to accomplish a task. Along these lines, one student reported that he "can't" study after 7pm because his medication has worn off and he is "fried." Although this might legitimately be the case, it is worth challenging his routine of not working after 7pm. One possible approach is to consider task list items that would be easier to do at this time of night. For example, it might be less mentally taxing to respond to e-mail or update your task list in the evening than to start writing the introduction to your term paper. Alternatively, some students have found that scheduling a study group or a tutor in the evening might provide the additional structure that they need to be able to focus at this time of day. The therapist will likely need to spend some time in session discussing how to get "un-stuck" from the routine of not working in the evenings (see Dialogue 3).

Dialogue 3

Therapist: Last week you told me that you can't study at night because you are too fried.

Client: Yes, I really need to take a break in the evenings because I am mentally exhausted.

Therapist: Is it working for you to take the evenings off? Do you feel refreshed after taking a break? Are you doing as well in your classes as you would like?

Client: No. It doesn't seem like there are enough hours in the day to do all the things on my list.

Therapist: Do you think things would be better if you were able to be productive in the evenings?

Client: Yes, but I don't think I can do it.

Therapist: Would you consider trying to re-arrange some of the things that you do so that you could use your evening time more productively for things that are less mentally challenging?

Client: What do you mean?

Therapist: Is there any chore that you routinely do in the mornings that doesn't require a lot of mental effort that you could move to the evenings so that you could do something more mentally challenging in the morning?

Client: I usually do my laundry on Friday mornings.

Therapist: Could you try doing your laundry on Thursday night this week so that you can do schoolwork on Friday morning?

Client: Yes, I think that might work. I will try it.

Discuss Homework and Follow-Up

This is the final planned session in this module, and as such, the end of session will look somewhat different from client to client. The therapist should first encourage students to continue to check and update their calendars and task lists on at least a daily basis, and to use the motivational techniques that were introduced last session. Students should also practice breaking down a task from their own list into smaller steps, with the intent of using this on an ongoing basis.

At this point, the therapist should have some reasonable idea as to whether the client immediately needs to complete an additional module or modules. If this has not been concretely discussed previously, the therapist should broach the topic of continuation (or termination) with each individual client.

- If there is agreement that an additional module is desirable at this time, make specific plans for a time and date to meet next, and give a brief overview of the content and rationale of the next module to instill further motivation to continue. Instruct the client on any materials that he or she might need for this next session, as well as any reading or other preparation that might be warranted.
- If you determine that the client's current issues have been adequately addressed or that the client is not motivated to continue active therapy at this time, schedule a "booster" session within the next 60 days to check in on continued proficiency in organization and time management (and other skills, if appropriate) and sustained functional gains, and to offer additional modules if warranted.
- Whether continuing or terminating with the client, the therapist is counseled to follow up with the client, either by phone or email, within the next week to answer questions and offer support in the implementation of OTMP skills taught in this module.

References

Knouse, L.E., & Mitchell, J.T. (2015). Incautiously optimistic: Positively valenced cognitive avoidance in adult ADHD. *Cognitive and Behavioral Practice, 22*(2), 192–202. 10.1016/j.cbpra.2014.06.003

Ramsay, J.R. (2016). "Turning intentions into actions": CBT for adult ADHD focused on implementation. *Clinical Case Studies, 15*(3), 179–197. 10.1177/1534650115611483

Ramsay, J.R., & Rostain, A.L. (2016). Adult attention-deficit/hyperactivity disorder as an implementation problem: Clinical significance, underlying mechanisms, and psychosocial treatment. *Practice Innovations, 1*(1), 36–52. https://doi-org.proxy006.nclive.org/10.1037/pri0000016

Strohmeier, C.W., Rosenfield, B., DiTomasso, R.A., & Ramsay, J.R. (2016). Assessment of the relationship between self-reported cognitive distortions and adult ADHD, anxiety, depression, and hopelessness. *Psychiatry Research, 238*, 153–158. https://doi-org.proxy006.nclive.org/10.1016/j.psychres.2016.02.034

Skill 2: Becoming a Professional Learner

(1–2 sessions)

Corresponds to Skillset 2 of the *Thriving in College* Student Workbook

Background for the Therapist

As noted in the OTMP module and elsewhere, the most inherent "job" of college students, with and without ADHD, is to succeed in their educational program and to earn their degree. Robust OTMP skills are critical in focusing students with ADHD on the tasks that they need to complete in this endeavor, but they are not specific to *the learning process itself* as it applies to learning information, understanding concepts, and demonstrating that learning on exams, papers, and projects. Having mastery of a complete set of academic skills—note taking in lectures and from readings, preparation for exams, and information- and help-seeking strategies—is also critical to success at the college level. Emerging empirical evidence suggests that many students with ADHD enter their undergraduate years with deficient academic skill preparation (Canu et al., 2021; DuPaul et al., 2021) and that academic skill deficits partially explain the relation between ADHD symptoms and poorer academic performance (Gormley et al., 2018). As such, educating this group regarding pertinent strategies and reinforcing and troubleshooting their efforts in implementation is an important treatment goal for many clients.

There are many strategies that students may use in effective studying, and individual differences exist in preferences and fit. However, we suggest that clinicians use one session to introduce college students with ADHD to a core set of academic skill strategies. Then, based on the size of the client's current skill repertoire and their need for additional support for implementation, the clinician and client(s) can focus on specific strategies as needed in subsequent sessions. Strategies in the module include:

1 Structuring work time and space to manage distractions (stay "in the zone")
2 Using effective learning and memory strategies
3 Taking notes effectively
4 Communicating with and seeking help from professors and peers

DOI: 10.4324/9781003149590-10

As with other modules in this intervention, these academic skills can be presented to students in a group, individual or combined individual-and-group therapy format. In practice, these skills are relatively speedy to introduce, but it is the successful *implementation* of the strategies by students that counts. We recommend that these academic skills be introduced in the course of one therapy session, but clinicians who use this approach may want to plan a second session or other follow-ups (i.e., in-between-sessions check-ins, or designated times during subsequent sessions that deliver other content) to ensure that clients are having success in implementing effective study habits. It also may be a good idea to "inject" this session and the academic skills material mid-therapy; as an example, you might find that doing sessions 1–3 of the *Organization, Time Management, and Planning Skills* could then be followed by *Academic Skills*, which would then naturally allow for some follow-up at OTMP session 4. In any event, the timing of follow-up should vary depending on the timing of introduction of these skills. For instance, if the *Educating Clients* and OTMP modules have been implemented in a Fall semester with a client (or set of clients), this module might be used at the beginning of the Spring term. In that case, follow-up might occur after two-to-four weeks in the Spring term have elapsed; however, it might then be good to employ check-ins on academic skills in other sessions (or follow-up contacts) again near midterm and finals, if possible.

For simplicity of presentation and implementation, we include one full session outline here that includes the didactic content for academic skills, per se. We also have included optional session materials, which can be utilized as part stand-alone skills reinforcement and also will be particularly helpful for students who may benefit from learning about and accessing academic or testing accommodations. Keep in mind that disability services resources are different at each institution and so you should gather information about the resources and procedures available at the student's school before presenting this session to them.

Generally speaking, while we suggest that Psychoeducation and OTMP are the core modules for intervention with college students with ADHD (i.e., *necessary* for their successful adaptation), this Academic Skills module will also be appropriate for *most* clients and should be implemented as early as possible to help students with ADHD avoid undue failure in their initial semester(s) in higher education.

Student Workbook

If you are using the *Thriving in College* student workbook, you will find that Skillset 2 on *Professional Learner Skills* corresponds to the material in this section. In this therapist guide, we recommend that you assess your client's specific needs for academic skills in Session 1 and tailor the content you emphasize accordingly. As such, Session 1 in the manual corresponds to multiple modules in the workbook, allowing you to tailor skills information and skills practice opportunities to each client.

Therapist Guide Session	Workbook Modules
1	2.0 Why it Matters, Pre-Assessment, and Roadmap
	2.1 Create Your Ideal Workspace
	2.2 Get In (and Stay In) the Focus Zone
	2.3 Power Studying with Successive Relearning
	2.4 Take Effective and Efficient Notes
2	2.5 Seek Help Effectively

References

Canu, W. H., Stevens, A. E., Ranson, L. M., Lefler, E. K., LaCount, P. A., Serrano, J. W., Willcutt, E., & Hartung, C. M. (2021). College readiness: Differences between first-year undergraduates with and without ADHD. *Journal of Learning Disabilities, 54*(6), 403–411. 10.1177/0022219420972693

DuPaul, G.J., Gormley, M.J., Anastopoulos, A.D., Weyandt, L.L., Labban, J., Sass, A.J., Busch, C.Z., Franklin, M.K., & Postler, K.B. (2021). Academic trajectories of college students with and without adhd: Predictors of four-year outcomes. *Journal of Clinical Child & Adolescent Psychology, 0*(0), 1–16. 10.1080/15374416.2020.1867990

Gormley, M.J., Pinho, T., Pollack, B., Puzino, K., Franklin, M.K., Busch, C., DuPaul, G.J., Weyandt, L.L., & Anastopoulos, A.D. (2018). Impact of study skills and parent education on first-year GPA among college students with and without ADHD. *Journal of Attention Disorders, 0*(0), 1087054715594422. 10.1177/1087054715594422

Session 1: Implement New Academic Skills

Corresponds to Modules 2.0–2.6 in the *Thriving in College* Student Workbook

Session Outline

1 Check-in with client(s)
2 Set agenda
3 Strategies to Increase Focus (Stay "In the Zone")
4 Effective Learning and Memory Strategies
5 Note-Taking Strategies
6 Getting Help from Professors
7 Getting Help from Peers
8 Discuss homework
9 Set time and date for the next meeting

Session Organization

Administration Format

As with many other sessions, this can be administered in a group or individual format. The group format may again be more desirable, for efficiency and also to facilitate peer encouragement and sharing of learning strategies that work.

Materials Needed

It is highly recommended that therapists bring copies of the *handouts* that both illustrate and outline the academic skills that are being taught in this session. While these skills are speedy for a therapist to introduce, it is still quite a lot of material to absorb, particularly for a student with ADHD. Having "take aways" that remind clients of the steps they will need to complete to implement academic strategies is essential. We have included a sample handout and worksheet in this section that can be copied and used by therapists for the academic skills we introduce here (see Appendix A), but therapists can feel free to create their own as they see fit.

DOI: 10.4324/9781003149590-11

Session Content

Check in with Client(s)

It is likely that clients have recently completed Psychoeducation and Organization, Time Management, and Planning sessions of this intervention, and as such may have questions or comments regarding that material. Check-in time can be used to solicit brief discussion, or simply to see how things are going and build rapport. In the event that this session is the first meeting with clients, check-in might focus more on feelings and expectations about therapy. In any event, aim for this to be brief (< 5 minutes), encouraging for any additional discussion of this sort to be postponed until after the session content is completed. We also recommend having your client complete the *Progress Tracker* (see Appendix B), and briefly touching base on any declines or improvements in school functioning.

Set Agenda

Introduce the agenda for this session to the client (see above). It may be helpful to have a visual aid to refer to, such as a flip chart or projected PowerPoint slide or printed handout. At this time, it might also be helpful to remind clients to write notes regarding important points in a therapy notebook. Setting the agenda should be speedily completed (< 2 minutes).

Strategies to Increase Focus (Stay "In the Zone")

This group of skills is aimed at reducing distractibility during less-than-stimulating schoolwork tasks by structuring the environment to reduce distractions and by structuring time and tasks to promote focus (the Pomodoro Technique).

Creating a Low-Distraction Study Environment

A common pitfall for college students, and particularly those with ADHD, is "studying" in environments that are more conducive to distraction than to concentration, like common spaces in dorms, shared bedrooms, and open, public spaces that are found in buildings like their university library or student union. While some can put on earbuds, tilt their head down, and focus on their study (or other academic work) materials, it is common for students to be frequently distracted and ineffective in such locations. In our experience, students with ADHD tend to have difficulty with these types of environments. Many students with ADHD who were successful enough in high school to progress to college may have had an appropriate, at-home space (e.g., a quiet, well-stocked desk or kitchen table) that was maintained and monitored by concerned parents for after-school study. As such, students may not have ever pondered or experimented with what kinds of environments work best for them in terms of promoting focused mental effort. This is their chance to get curious and creative about the environments that can best support them.

Engage the client in a discussion of what kinds of stimuli are most likely to distract them when trying to focus on their schoolwork (see Dialogue 1 for an example). Also, see the list of possible distractions in Box 1 which may be helpful in guiding conversation. In our experience, the "best" choice of study environment can be quite specific to the individual student. For example, some students prefer complete silence when studying while others find total silence aversive and prefer low-intensity background noise or lyric-free music. Interestingly, some limited research suggests that people with ADHD may be more likely to benefit cognitively from background music or "white noise" (Abikoff et al., 1996; Söderlund et al., 2007), but there are substantial individual differences in these effects (Pelham et al., 2011).

Dialogue 1

Therapist: *Where do you usually study?*

Client: *I like to study in my dorm room.*

Therapist: *Do you have a desk that you sit at in your room?*

Client: *Yes, but I prefer to sit on my bed with my laptop on my lap.*

Therapist: *How does this work for you?*

Client: *It works okay. It's comfortable.*

Therapist: *Are you productive when you sit down to work?*

Client: *Sometimes but I don't think it is related to where I am studying. I think that I would have trouble concentrating no matter where I was.*

Therapist: *Would it be okay with you if we talked through this a bit more to try to determine why you are not always as productive as you would like to be?*

Client: *Sure.*

Therapist: *Tell me more about what happens when you sit down on your bed to start studying or dome homework.*

Client: *I get all my stuff out that I think I am going to need and then I fill up my water bottle. Once I sit down, I try to figure out what I will do first but sometimes I spend a bit of time on my phone first.*

Therapist: *Okay. Once you choose a task to get started on, what happens?*

Client: *Usually, I work on it for awhile, like maybe 10 or 20 minutes, and then I get distracted by something and decide to take a break.*

Therapist: *What are some examples of things you might get distracted by?*

Client: *Well, my roommate might come home and start talking to me or I hear other people out in the common area watching sports and I decide to go see what the score is.*

Therapist:	*How many hours do you think it takes you to complete one hour's worth of work?*
Client:	*It probably takes at least two hours because I get distracted and take breaks.*
Therapist:	*I wonder what would happen if you went to the library for one hour, finished one hour's worth of work, and then came home to relax in your dorm room or watch sports in the common room?*
Client:	*I don't like the idea of going to the library but it might be more productive and less frustrating.*
Therapist:	*Would you be willing to try it once this week?*
Client:	*Yes.*
Therapist:	*Would it be okay if we picked out a time now for you to try it?*
Client:	*Yes.* (Opens calendar on phone.) *It might work to go right after class tomorrow for one hour before I go home for dinner.*
Therapist:	*Great. I appreciate your willingness to try something new. If the library doesn't work for you, we can brainstorm some other ideas next week.*

Box 1   Possible distractions when trying to focus on schoolwork

Sound/noise: anything other than complete silence; complete silence distracts me; people talking, people whispering, music with lyrics; any music; noises that follow a rhythmic pattern (e.g., water dripping), alerts coming from my phone/laptop

Sights/visual: phone/laptop notifications, TV screens, people in the room, lights that are too bright, fluorescent lights

Comfort/Discomfort: uncomfortable seat, lack of writing surface, too hot/too cold

Devices: phone, laptop, TV, clock, specific apps or websites

Other humans: friends, off-task people

Emotions: feeling confused, feeling tired, feeling anxious

Thoughts: remembering something else I need to do; worry thoughts; thoughts about something I'd rather be doing

What keeps you in the zone? Coffee, having taken my medication, feeling like I'm accomplishing goals, I need really (inspiring/chill) music, other people around me working and on task, making a checklist of small steps and ticking them off as I get things done

Following a discussion of the most problematic distractions, engage the client in some troubleshooting, including identifying study locations with the most potential for supporting their focus. The list in Box 2 below gives sample suggestions for distraction management techniques. For locations, private study carrels are available in many college and university libraries and are often situated in quiet floors or areas. Some clients will benefit from establishing or rearranging their dorm or home desk area. Other students find that they focus best outside of their living (and sleeping!) space. Students with ADHD might investigate signing up for a personal study room, or scope out where such a space is available. Academic buildings on college campuses often have seating areas that are open, yet largely deserted after class hours are finished. Clients can ask their peers about treasured locations for optimal studying, both on campus and in the community. Students might be resistant to the idea of changing their study space, but therapists can explore the advantages and disadvantages of giving this a try and simply invite students to experiment with new locations.

Conclude this discussion by inviting the client to identify at least two new study locations and the "set up" for studying in that location – that is, what they will need to do to promote focus, such as cueing up an ambient music playlist or zipping their phone inside the pocket of their backpack. Homework related to this skill could include the client trying out their new study locations and strategies.

Box 2 Distraction-management techniques

Distracting noises: study in the silent section of the library; wear noise-canceling headphones and listen to lyric-free music (e.g., film soundtracks).

Sights/visual: keep all screens (phone, TVs, computer monitors) out of sight

Comfort/discomfort: make sure I'm warm enough; don't study in bed because I'll fall asleep; study at a desk only

Devices: only study with devices completely turned off; remove apps that are key distractions; turn off app and email notifications on laptop; set a timer so I don't have to keep checking the clock

Other humans: study alone; study alongside a friend who's good at staying on task; study at a coffee shop or at the library where others are on task

Emotions: set a specific goal for the work period, read directions twice; do a short mindfulness / deep breathing exercise before getting started

Thoughts: write a quick note to myself for later if I think of something I need to do; tell myself I can do a "rather be doing" thing later if I finish my work

The Pomodoro Technique

Educate your client about the Pomodoro method for reducing distractions and staying in the "study zone." Cirillo (2006) developed the Pomodoro Technique in college because he felt like he was wasting too much time when trying to study. In an effort to determine if he could study for 10 minutes straight without getting distracted, he pulled out a kitchen timer that was shaped like a tomato. ("Pomodoro" is the Italian word for "tomato"). Eventually, Cirillo developed the Pomodoro Technique and has trained others to use it to improve their work efficiency. The Pomodoro Technique involves working for 25 minutes at a time and then taking a break. Cirillo recommends the following pattern:

1st pomodoro: Work for 25 minutes
1st break: Take a 3- to 5-minute break
2nd pomodoro: Work for 25 minutes
2nd break: Take a 3- to 5-minute break
3rd pomodoro: Work for 25 minutes
3rd break: Take a 3- to 5-minute break
4th pomodoro: Work for 25 minutes
4th break: Take a 15- to 30-minute break

This entire cycle will take 2 to 2 ½ hours depending on the length of breaks. Cirillo provided some additional guidelines for preventing distraction during each pomodoro. First, clients should be strict with themselves about not allowing interruptions during pomodoros. Clients should keep a paper and pen nearby. If they have a thought about something else that needs to be dealt with, they should make a note for later and get back to work. Second, if a pomodoro is interrupted by something out of the client's control (e.g., another person, a need to go to the bathroom, a fire drill), then that pomodoro is void and they should start over once the interruption has subsided. This is meant to increase motivation to avoid interruptions so that progress toward a longer break is not hindered. Third, when the timer goes off, the client must take a break even if they are tempted to continue their work. They should at least walk around the room, stretch or get a drink of water before starting the next pomodoro. Clients should avoid doing anything mentally challenging or stressful during a break (e.g., making work-related phone calls, returning e-mails), as the quality of the break may impact productivity during the next pomodoro. Fourth, during the longer break, clients might be able to take care of some tasks that are not particularly mentally challenging (e.g., get coffee, chat with a friend, check Facebook, watch a 20-minute show on Netflix). Once the client has completed a four-pomodoro cycle, Cirillo recommends starting additional cycles until major goals for the day are complete. Finally, clients can adjust the length of pomodoros and breaks, within reason. Cirillo (2006) indicated that pomodoros will be most effective if they last from 20 to 45 minutes; thus, the recommended starting point of 25 minutes can be adjusted based on personal preference. We have found several apps that help individuals use the Pomodoro Technique while simultaneously discouraging use of the internet and social media. Some of the apps are exclusively for mobile phones; some, like Flat Tomato, Repeat Timer, Tomato Timer, and Block and Flow are freely available, whereas more gamified (and maybe more motivating) versions like Forest are available at low cost. Other apps can be used on a computer, such as Pomodor (free!). Please note that these particular apps were available at the time that this manual was written, but some may no longer be available. We are confident, though, that searching the iPhone or Android app store for pomodoro timers or productivity apps (e.g., SelfControl, StayFocusd) will yield options that you can refer clients to.

Effective Learning and Memory Strategies

This set of skills includes three main strategies: self-testing, distributed practice, and mnemonics. Educate the client about each strategy, emphasizing that each is based upon what we know from psychology "works" for long-lasting learning (Dunlosky et al., 2013). In preparing students to learn these techniques, it is important to inform them that these strategies will *feel* more difficult and effortful than less effective learning strategies, a phenomenon referred to as *desirable difficulty* (Bjork, 1994). Educate your client that, although these strategies may feel "harder" or like they are not working, the effort they put in during the learning process is likely to pay off later in terms of better retention.

Self-Testing

Self-testing involves repeatedly attempting to retrieve information from memory when trying to learn material. Most students quiz themselves to try to determine *what* they know, but the act of trying to remember itself has powerful effects on the likelihood of remembering information in the future. In particular, self-testing results in superior memory compared to simple restudy methods like re-reading textbook chapters or looking over study guides, regardless of whether students have ADHD (Knouse et al., 2016); however, people with ADHD may be less likely to use or stick with self-testing strategies (Knouse et al., 2012).

The most common way that students use self-testing to study is probably by using **flashcards** – either physical or digital; however, there are many more ways that students can self-test in order to achieve better memory for important information (see Box 3). Encourage the client to think about self-testing more broadly. Any method that requires them to pull information from memory can count!

When using flashcards specifically, the way the cards are used matters. Clients should keep two methods in mind.

- Students **should not simply re-read** the answers over and over. Cards should be formatted in such a way that they can look at the prompt before revealing the answer. Students should try their best to **think of the answer themselves** before flipping the card over. Even unsuccessful recall attempts can strengthen memory.
- Students should typically not "drop" a card or study item after just one correct recall attempt. Studies show that making more than one successful recall attempt in a study session results in better memory. **Three correct recalls** is a good rule of thumb to use before dropping an item (Rawson & Dunlosky, 2011).

Next, ask clients to brainstorm other ways they could test or quiz themselves using their class materials, offering suggestions from Box 3. Help clients narrow down one or two new self-testing strategies they might want to try out in the coming week and help them plan which materials they will study and when.

Box 3   Ideas for Self-Testing While Studying

1   Make and study paper flash cards (be sure to put prompt and answer on opposite sides)
2   Use flashcard and quizzing apps to study (e.g., Quizlet)[1]
3   Complete reading quiz questions at the end of textbook sections and chapters
4   Draw important diagrams or concept maps from memory
5   Write down everything you can remember about a concept or reading assignment
6   Use the fold-over note page method (see section on Two-Column note-taking, below)
7   In a small study group, quiz each other on to-be-learned information
8   Call your parent or grandparent and tell them what you learned in class that day
9   Explain the main ideas of a reading assignment to your roommate

---

Distributed Practice

Most college students have probably heard at some point that "cramming" is not the best way to study, and scientific literature strongly supports this notion (Dunlosky et al., 2013). Distributed practice, or spacing out study sessions over time, is generally more effective than studying material all at once (massed practice). When students cram, they are also likely to be highly stressed or sleep-deprived and these conditions have their own negative effects on memory and learning. Discuss with students how spacing out their study sessions will result in better learning and probably also lower their stress levels as well.

Combining distributed practice with self-testing results in the powerful strategy of **successive re-learning** (Rawson et al., 2018) or **repeated re-learning**. Research suggests that studying material using self-testing three or four sessions with a day or two in between results in strong effects on memory (Rawson & Dunlosky, 2011). In a single session, students should study material using self-testing and continue until they can correctly recall each piece of information at least three times. The next time they approach this same material, it is likely to take less time to hit this learning mark, meaning that later sessions will be shorter and less burdensome. Finally, students can, of course, self-test again right before the test for maximum short term recall boost. To manage the timing of these sessions, students can schedule study times in their calendars in advance of scheduled quizzes or exams. As described above, work with your client to schedule specific times for studying using self-testing in their calendar.

Mnemonics

College-level concepts tend to be more complex and the *quantity* of information that one is expected to learn is often much greater. Mnemonics are a memory strategy often introduced in elementary school (e.g., "Roy G. Biv" for the colors of the light wave spectrum) and mnemonics continue to have relevance for college material. A mnemonic creates a cue to remember a set of information and allows one to "chunk" or make added associations for knowledge and thereby retrieve it from memory more easily. There are several types of mnemonics (for example, see Congos, 2006, https://www.learningassistance.com/2006/january/mnemonics.html), and there are probably an infinite number of possible mnemonics for the variety of information one might want to learn, allowing students to find the most useful format for their own learning and memory styles. Several common types of mnemonics are described in Box 4 below.

Box 4   Common Types of Mnemonics

Word (or expression) mnemonics. Helpful for remembering lists. The first letter of each item in the list is used as a letter in a mnemonic word (e.g., "FANBOYS" for the coordinating conjunctions of the English language) or expression (e.g., "Please Excuse My Dear Aunt Sally" for the order of mathematical operations).

Name mnemonics. A variation of the word mnemonic. First letters of a list of items can be arranged into a memorable name, for example, "Pvt. Tim Hall," for the essential amino acids.

Music mnemonics. Students can create songs that encompass details of academic information that they want to remember. Incredibly long lists can be memorized in this way (e.g., the "Countries of the World" song from the *Animaniacs* animated series).

Model mnemonics. Particularly helpful for visual learners, conceptual information can often be depicted in a model, for example, the pyramidal Maslow's Hierarchy of Needs.

Image mnemonics. Visual cues for memory can be particularly powerful. For example, in the method of loci, a learner imagines concepts or words as objects that appear along a path that they have frequently traveled. Remember, the list of concepts is then a matter of mentally traveling the path and listing off the items that appear along the way. Simpler image mnemonics combine verbal and visual cues. For instance, if trying to remember names of depressant drugs – barbiturates, alcohol, and tranquilizers – you might think of the word "BAT," and visualizing a bat, complete with drooping wings and a "frowny" face, signifying the depressant feature of these drugs. The more unusual and visually rich the image, the more memorable it will be.

In addition to the ones described in Box 4, there are a variety of other memory techniques that could be described as mnemonic in nature, and it is somewhat beyond the scope of this manual to review them all. Discuss with your client which kinds of strategies they would like to try out for which material in the coming week.

Note-Taking Strategies

Two-Column Method of Notetaking

This method is based on the well-known Cornell Notetaking Method (Pauk & Owens, 2010) and can be used for taking notes from readings or from lectures. The student should draw a line lengthwise down the page to create a left column

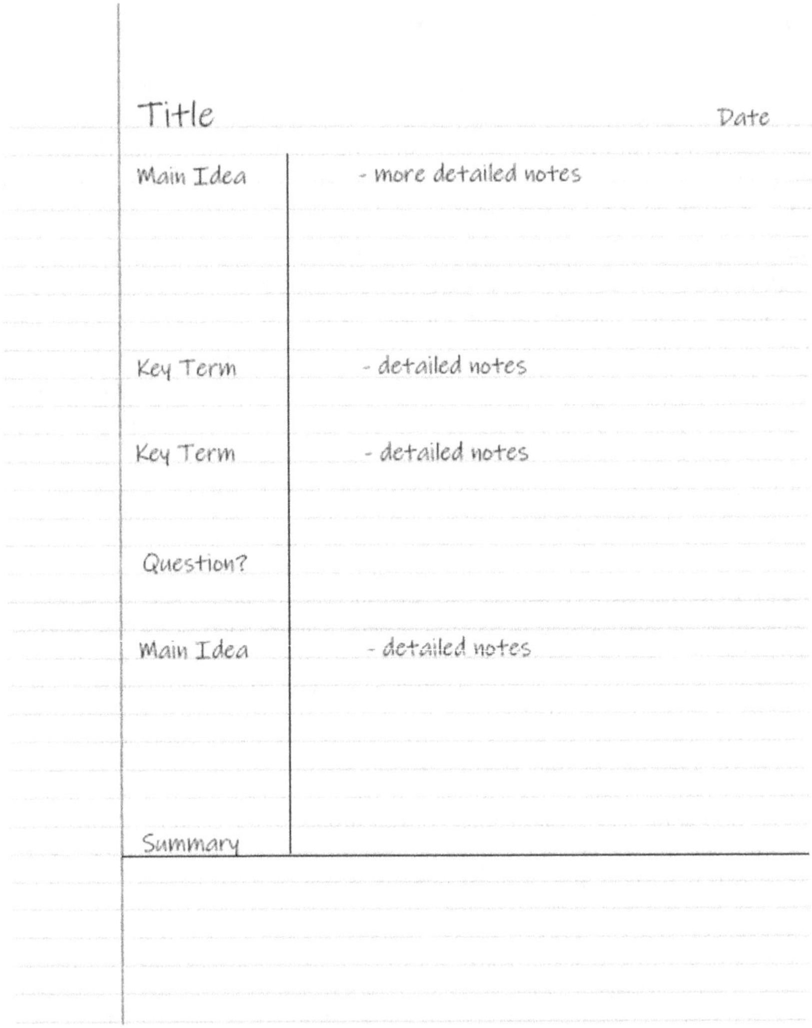

```
 |
 |  Title                                        Date
 |─────────────────┬──────────────────────────────────
 |  Main Idea      │  - more detailed notes
 |                 │
 |                 │
 |                 │
 |                 │
 |  Key Term       │  - detailed notes
 |                 │
 |  Key Term       │  - detailed notes
 |                 │
 |                 │
 |  Question?      │
 |                 │
 |  Main Idea      │  - detailed notes
 |                 │
 |                 │
 |                 │
 |  Summary        │
 |─────────────────┴──────────────────────────────────
 |
 |
 |
```

Figure 1 Example Format for Two Column Method of Notetaking.

that is about ⅓ of the page (See Figure 1). The student should record their **more detailed notes in the larger right column** and put corresponding **main ideas or keywords in the left column**. For the main notes section, bullet points work best rather than complete sentences. Finally, students can add a summary at the bottom of each page to help consolidate what they've learned.

When reading a chapter in a textbook, students can list the topic headers and main ideas in the left column and add more detailed notes to the right column.

In some situations, students may want to identify one main idea per paragraph. For other readings, they may want to choose one main idea per page, section or chapter. However, it should be noted that not all paragraphs or pages have new main ideas, and that certain types of readings (e.g., novels, short stories, or biographies) will require some alertness on the student's part in terms of identifying main sections, themes, and important points, as these may not have clear or any headings, depending on their specific nature.

When listening to a lecture, students will again list the main ideas or important concepts in the left column and the details in the right column. If the lecturer is using presentation slides, students may be able to identify one main idea and multiple details per slide. If there are no slides, then students will need to pay closer attention to the lecture in order to identify the main ideas and important concepts.

During the session, model and have the client practice this note taking method using a reading example and a lecture example. For the lecture example, you could "formally" present information regarding the two-column notes method, using the details above. Alternatively, you could find a suitable lecture video on the internet, and play a five-minute segment for this exercise. For the reading example, you could choose a few paragraphs from a General Psychology or Abnormal Psychology textbook and prepare an example in advance. Choose a few paragraphs that have relatively clear main ideas and supporting details to create the most useful example for modeling.

Importantly, students can easily **use two-column notes for self-testing** by folding the page along the line dividing the left and right columns, looking at the main idea or key word column, and attempting to recall the supporting details before checking their responses. Content from the columns can also be used to create flashcards.

Getting Help from Professors

When students transition from high school to college, they need to adapt to the often-mysterious norms of higher education academia. Without specific instruction, some students may not understand how to most effectively get help from their professors or teaching assistants, that they *can* request assistance, or even that they can and should ask for help when they need it also while taking advantage of the resources provided by the instructor for self-help. Discuss with the client their experiences requesting and receiving help from instructors and offer help with the skills described below.

Use Resources Provided by the Instructor

In other words, students should always **check the syllabus** as the first step for questions about the course. In our experience, students can quickly forget that this document typically provides a course schedule with reading assignments, a summary of course policies, and other key information. We recommend that, at the start

---

Box 5   Have a question about something in your class? Don't wonder! Follow these steps:

- Check the syllabus for the answer to your question
- Visit the course page online [Blackboard, Canvas, Moodle] for the answer to your question
- Carefully reread the instructions for the assignment for the answer
- Go to your instructor's weekly office hours to ask your question or ask for help
- If none of the above answer your questions, email your professor or teaching assistant

---

of each semester, students **enter all the key dates and assignments due dates from the syllabus into their calendar system**. While not every instructor puts detailed and helpful information in their syllabus, many do and checking here first can eliminate unnecessary back-and-forth via email. Students should also take time to become familiar with information on the **course learning management system (LMS)**, if applicable. Common online LMS platforms include Canvas, Blackboard, and Moodle and these resources often include a course calendar, assignments, course readings, and a gradebook. Finally, students should be encouraged to **carefully read assignment instructions** before they get started on an assignment and to revisit these instructions frequently while completing the assignment to make sure they are on track. Students should **take advantage of weekly office hours**, when instructors are ready and waiting (often alone!) to help them and answer their questions. Visiting office hours in the first two weeks of the semester just to introduce yourself can be a great way to connect with a professor, especially in a large class. The more professors get to know their students, the easier it is to provide help to them when needed (See Box 5).

Address Instructors Appropriately

Discuss with clients that they are more likely to get what they need from instructors if the instructor feels respected and valued (this is true for most people, not just professors!). Academic titles, such as "Dr." and "Professor" are one way that accomplishment and status are acknowledged in a college setting. Unfortunately, we have observed that some instructors are less likely to be afforded these titles of respect than others – for example, students are less likely to initially address women, younger instructors, or people of color as "Dr." or

"Professor," and some studies support this observation (Rubin, 1981; Takiff et al., 2001). Especially if you are working with clients who are just starting college, discuss with them that the best policy is to **call their instructor "Dr." or "Professor" and their last name, unless otherwise instructed.** This way, students ensure that they are applying these honorific titles to their instructors and showing respect regardless of age, race, or gender identity. As a result, they are more likely to form a favorable impression with the instructor and start their relationship on the right foot.

Effective Email Communication with Instructors

During our 60+ years collective experience as university-level instructors, we have noted several trends in communication from students that therapists might watch out for and focus on in working with college student clients. First, many students do not use clear or professional communication with instructors or teaching assistants. Second, students do not take full advantage of the resources that might answer their questions, such as those mentioned in the previous section (e.g., office hours, syllabus, LMS). Third, student questions and requests often arrive too late for the instructor to be helpful, such as the night before a test or major assignment due date. Discuss with the clients how they typically get help and information in their classes and review the following principles for communication with instructors. It is important to frame these guidelines as **methods for helping the client get what they want and need from instructors** as opposed to simply adhering to meaningless norms of conduct. In addition, clear and professional communication is a very important professional skill for the student's life after college!

Because much out-of-class communication with instructors occurs via email, we tend to focus on that mode of communication with our student clients. Figure 2 summarizes this approach.

Writing Effective Emails to Professors: Just Remember DEAR* PROF!

Describe: describe the current situation

"I was invited to interview for Teach for America; however, the interview is scheduled for the same day as our exam."

Explain: explain your perspective on the situation

"I am concerned, since this is the only interview day and I will be unable to take the exam on the day it has been scheduled."

Ask: clearly and specifically ask for what you want

"Therefore, I am wondering if you would please consider allowing me to take the exam two days early."

Reward: explain positive consequences and "what's in it for them"

"I can be available to work around your schedule. Thank you, in advance, for your help."

PROFessional: helpful subject line; address professor appropriately; greet and close

"Subject: taking the Intro Psychology exam early"

"Dear Dr. Jones,"

"Sincerely, Jon"

Be sure to email a day or two **in advance** so that they have sufficient time to respond.

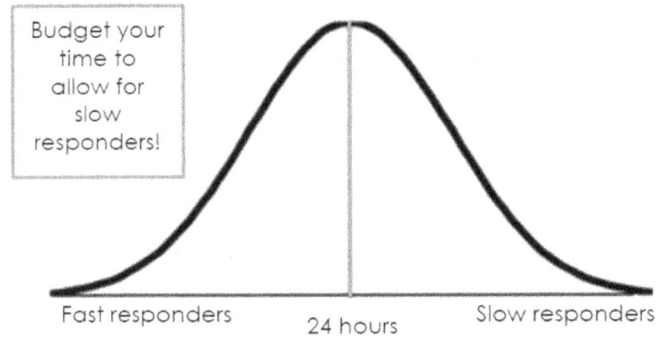

Figure 2 The DEAR PROF strategy for writing emails to professors.
*Adapted from *DBT Skills Training Manual* by Marsha Linehan (2014).

As illustrated in Figure 2, the approach to effective communication with professors is modeled on content from Marsha Linehan's *DBT Skills Training* in Interpersonal Effectiveness (Linehan, 2014). In addition to outlining a method for clear communication, these steps create a handy "DEAR Prof" mnemonic (see description of this memory technique above) to help students remember the steps for writing an effective email.

The content of the message is specified in the acronym "DEAR." Students should first **describe** the relevant circumstances in a "just the facts" manner. Next, preferably on a new line, they should **explain** (or express) their feelings, perspectives, or concerns – that is, state the purpose of the communication. Next – and perhaps most importantly – students should clearly **ask** for what they want from the professor. Many student emails lack a clear "ask," which leaves the instructor unsure about how best to respond. Invite clients to suggest solutions to the problems they pose in their emails. Finally, students should indicate what will **reinforce** or reward the instructor for granting the request. Often, this can simply be an expression of thanks for considering the request.

"Prof" is short for "professional" and describes how the message should be framed. Here, professional framing includes addressing the recipient respectfully with the appropriate title, using a greeting and closing, and providing a descriptive and helpful subject line that indicates which class the student is enrolled in. Finally, as indicated in Figure 2, students should be encouraged to allow sufficient time for professors to respond. 24 hours is a reasonable expectation for an email response but if the student does not receive a response in that time frame, they should feel free to send a quick and polite reminder.

Getting Help from Peers

Communicating with Classmates

While fewer issues regarding professionalism apply to communication with classmates, clear communication with peers may be crucial when a student:

✓ *Misses class (or part of class)*
✓ *Has an upcoming exam*
✓ *Has a group project*

Obtaining Notes for Missed Classes

Whenever a student misses a class period, the student should **get class notes from a classmate**, even if class lecture outlines are made available by the professor. Missing class is never desirable and this is particularly true for students with ADHD who may benefit from in-person and auditory learning modalities. However, promptly getting notes from a peer can help mitigate negative consequences. For many clients, requesting notes from a classmate will require stepping out of their comfort zone. You should clearly convey to clients with ADHD, however, that any discomfort they experience will be worth it. The "DEAR" format for making effective requests may be useful here. Obtaining notes from a peer not only allows the client to double-check that they have all the material conveyed by the professor (which might ultimately be on an exam) but also to make sure that they are aware of any announcements made by the professor. If notes are unclear, the student should check with the peer for clarification first, and if concepts are still unclear, the student can approach the professor (or a course's graduate teaching assistant) after class or during office hours for help.

Studying with Peers

Peers can be excellent resources in preparing for examinations – especially if group studying involves testing each other on the material and teaching each other tough concepts. The first step for students with ADHD is to ask classmates if they are willing to meet to study together and, as above, "DEAR" skills may help reluctant students to frame these requests. Clients should be sure to put the scheduled session in their calendar, to send reminders to their group members, and to bring all needed materials to the session. For exams that cover a wide amount of information, group members can put more individual preparation focus on different portions of the required material, and then be responsible for leading the group review for that section of the material. Clients might also be reminded to thank their classmates for doing a group study session, which might encourage their peers to do it again.

Managing Group Projects

Group projects are common in college-level coursework. Effective communication between team members is vital. Students with ADHD could be advised that for highest efficacy this includes (a) agreeing on the topic and/or approach to the paper or presentation early in the work, (b) clearly communicating the division of labor, (c) setting clear individual goals for work between meetings and checking on progress toward goals regularly, (d) sharing relevant notes and information that could help others with their parts, and (e) making sure to schedule a practice session if a presentation is involved.

Discuss Homework and Set the Next Meeting

Five broad topics for improving academic performance were presented in this session:

- Strategies to Increase Focus (Stay "In the Zone")
- Effective Learning and Memory Strategies
- Note-Taking Strategies
- Getting Help from Professors
- Getting Help from Peers

Students should choose at least two new strategies to try this week and complete the handout (see Appendix A) so that they can track and share experiences with these strategies in the group or with their therapist at a subsequent session. Finally, make sure that you specifically note with the client(s) what day, time, and place the next session will be, optimally making sure that this is entered in his/her/their calendar(s).

References

Abikoff, H., Courtney, M.E., Szeibel, P.J., & Koplewicz, H.S. (1996). The effects of auditory stimulation on the arithmetic performance of children with adhd and nondisabled children. *Journal of Learning Disabilities, 29*(3), 238–246. 10.1177/002221949602900302

Bjork, R.A. (1994). Memory and metamemory considerations in the training of human beings. In J. Metcalfe & A.P. Shimamura (Eds.), *Metacognition: Knowing about Knowing* (pp. 185–205). MIT Press.

Cirillo, F. (2006). The Pomodoro Technique. *Currency.*

Congos, D. (2006). 9 Types of Mnemonics for Better Memory. *The Learning Center Exchange.*

Dunlosky, J., Rawson, K.A., Marsh, E.J., Nathan, M.J., & Willingham, D.T. (2013). Improving students' learning with effective learning techniques: Promising directions from cognitive and educational psychology. *Psychological Science in the Public Interest, 14*(1), 4–58. 10.1177/1529100612453266

Knouse, L.E., Anastopoulos, A.D., & Dunlosky, J. (2012). Isolating metamemory deficits in the self-regulated learning of adults with ADHD. *Journal of Attention Disorders, 16,* 650–660. 10.1177/1087054711417231

Knouse, L.E., Rawson, K.A., Vaughn, K.E., & Dunlosky, J. (2016). Does testing improve learning for college students with Attention-Deficit/Hyperactivity Disorder? *Clinical Psychological Science, 4*(1), 136–143. 10.1177/2167702614565175

Linehan, M.M. (2014). *DBT skills training manual* (2nd ed.). Guilford Press.

Pauk, W., Owens, R.J.Q. (2010). How to Study in College (10 ed.). *Boston, MA: Wadsworth.* (pp. 235–277). ISBN 978-1-4390-8446-5

Pelham, W.E., Waschbusch, D.A., Hoza, B., Gnagy, E.M., Greiner, A.R., Sams, S.E., Vallano, G., Majumdar, A., & Carter, R.L. (2011). Music and video as distractors for boys with adhd in the classroom: Comparison with controls, individual differences, and medication effects. *Journal of Abnormal Child Psychology, 39*(8), 1085–1098. 10.1007/s10802-011-9529-z

Rawson, K.A., & Dunlosky, J. (2011). Optimizing schedules of retrieval practice for durable and efficient learning: How much is enough? *Journal of Experimental Psychology: General, 140*(3), 283–302. 10.1037/a0023956

Rawson, K.A., Vaughn, K.E., Walsh, M., & Dunlosky, J. (2018). Investigating and explaining the effects of successive relearning on long-term retention. *Journal of Experimental Psychology: Applied, 24*(1), 57–71. 10.1037/xap0000146

Rubin, R.B. (1981). Ideal traits and terms of address for male and female college professors. *Journal of Personality and Social Psychology, 41*(5), 966–974. 10.1037/0022-3514.41.5.966

Söderlund, G., Sikström, S., & Smart, A. (2007). Listen to the noise: Noise is beneficial for cognitive performance in ADHD. *Journal of Child Psychology and Psychiatry, 48*(8), 840–847. 10.1111/j.1469-7610.2007.01749.x

Takiff, H.A., Sanchez, D.T., & Stewart, T.L. (2001). What's in a Name? The Status Implications of Students' Terms of Address for Male and Female Professors. *Psychology of Women Quarterly, 25*(2), 134–144. 10.1111/1471-6402.00015

Session 2: Follow-up and Academic Support and Accommodations

Corresponds to Module 2.6 in the *Thriving in College* Student Workbook

Session Outline

1 Check-in with client(s)
2 Set agenda
3 Review academic skills homework
4 Provide psychoeducation about accommodations
5 Discuss which accommodations and campus resources might be helpful
6 Discuss homework
7 Set time and date for next meeting

Session Organization

Administration Format

This session can be administered in a group or individual format.

Materials Needed

It is highly recommended that therapists bring copies of *handouts* that present and summarize information being taught in this session. We have included sample handouts that can be copied and used by therapists for the academic skills we introduce here (see Appendix A), but therapists can feel free to create their own as they see fit. In addition, if discussing possible disability accommodations, students should bring to the session any *assessment reports or other relevant educational or clinical documentation* that might establish their ADHD as a disability and that might provide clues to helpful accommodations for that disability.

Session Content

Check-in with Client(s)

It is unlikely that this will be the first technique or content-heavy session that a client has done with you. Check-in time can be used to solicit brief discussion, or

DOI: 10.4324/9781003149590-12

simply to see how things are going and build rapport. In the event that this session is the first meeting with clients, check-in might focus more on feelings and expectations about therapy. In any event, aim for this to be brief (< 5 minutes), encouraging for any additional discussion of this sort to be postponed until after the session content is completed. See therapist-client check-in dialogue example in Skill 1: Session 1 as a model for this interaction, if needed. We also recommend having your client complete the *Progress Tracker* (see Appendix B), and briefly touching base on any declines or improvements in school functioning.

Set Agenda

Introduce the agenda for this session to the client (see Session Outline). It may be helpful to have a visual aid to refer to, such as a flip chart or projected PowerPoint slide or printed handout. At this time, it might also be helpful to remind clients to write notes regarding important points in a therapy notebook. Setting the agenda should be speedily completed (< 2 minutes).

Review and Troubleshoot the Academic Skills Homework

Using the Academic Skills Homework sheet from the prior session, if available, review the client's skill practice goals including what worked and what needs to be modified. Be sure to enthusiastically praise any change attempts. For skills that did not work as well as they could, ask questions to determine how the client tried to implement the skill and whether there are ways they could modify the use of the skill to work better. If clients did not engage in academic skills practice, discuss how they can remind and motivate themselves to do so next week using the skills learned in the OTMP module. Finally, work with the client to identify two repeat or new academic skills to work on in the coming week using the handout from the previous session. We also recommend having your client complete the *Progress Tracker* (see Appendix B), and briefly touching base on any declines or improvements in school functioning.

Provide Psychoeducation about Academic Accommodations in College

Even if they received special education services in high school, many clients with ADHD may not be informed about academic accommodations in college and how to get them.

First, ask the client what they know about accommodations in college and fill in any gaps in their knowledge. If the client received special education services in high school, it may be helpful to specifically educate them about the differences between special education services in K-12 education and accommodations for people with disabilities in college, which are provided under the Americans with Disabilities Act (ADA; see Table 1).

Table 1 Comparison of Special Education Services and Accommodations under the Americans with Disabilities Act (ADA)

	K-12	*Higher Education*
Main applicable law	Individuals with Disabilities in Education Act (IDEA) – an education law	Americans with Disabilities Act (ADA) – a civil rights law
Goal of accommodation	Maximize educational **success** for students with disabilities	Provide equal **access** to educational activities and settings for people with disabilities
Who identifies the need for services?	The school system	The student
Who must obtain and pay for documentation and testing to determine eligibility?	The school system	The student
Key document	Individualized Education Plan (IEP)	Letter of Accommodation (LOA) or Disability Accommodation Notice (DAN)
Can the curriculum and standards be modified?	Yes – content of what is taught and expectations may be individualized to the student	No – content of what is taught and performance standards do not change
Is access to specialized instruction guaranteed?	Yes – if the student's IEP includes it	No – but many schools offer tutoring or other academic skills support to all students

Explain that:

1 Accommodations are provided based on determination of **a documented disability**: a physical or mental impairment that substantially limits one or more major life activities, and,
2 The goal of accommodations under the ADA is not to ensure academic *success*; rather it is to **provide equal *access*** to the classroom, learning materials, and assessments.

For example, providing a person with ADHD with a quiet environment in which to take a test does not ensure that they will get a good grade, but rather allows that person an equal opportunity to demonstrate their knowledge on the test (Gordon et al., 2015).

Discuss which Accommodations Might Be Helpful

Next, engage the client in a discussion of testing and learning situations where their ADHD symptoms get in the way and where accommodations may be useful (see example in Dialogue 1). Review with them any assessment reports or other documentation for records of accommodations received or clinical recommendations that might point toward useful accommodations. Importantly, **requested accommodations should not change what is taught or what is expected in terms of the student's performance** but, again, the goal is to provide equal access to the learning experiences and materials offered in the student's course of study compared to their peers.

Importantly, no accommodation has been demonstrated to specifically "level the playing field" for all students with ADHD and, in some cases, accommodations may have little impact or even detrimental impact on performance (Miller et al., 2015; Weis & Beauchemin, 2020). As such, encourage the student to **think carefully about whether each accommodation would actually improve access for them,** rather than just going with what they have typically received or what they are accustomed to. Their needs may have changed since high school!

Common academic accommodation for students with ADHD include:

1 **Testing Accommodations:** additional time to complete exams[1], permission to complete exams in a quiet space, permission to type answers on a computer instead of hand-writing them
2 **Classroom Accommodations**: permission to audio record lectures, access to a note-taker, class notes, and/or lecturer's lesson plan or slides
3 **Learning Material Accommodations**: Access to audio versions of textbooks or screen readers

Discuss Other Academic Support Services

In addition to accommodations based on a disability determination, many college campuses have substantial resources available to all students for help in developing their academic and self-management skills. Engage the client in a discussion of which of these resources they might access and what may be helpful, including:

- Individual or group tutoring (Academic Skills Center)
- Academic and time management skill assessments and coaching (Academic Skills Center)
- Writing instruction and coaching (Writing Center)
- Public speaking and presentation coaching (Speech Center)
- Assistance with identifying library and scholarly resources (Librarians or Reference desk)

Dialogue 1

Therapist: You mentioned a couple of sessions ago that you had testing or classroom accommodations in the past in school. Tell me a little bit more about that.

Client: Yeah, in high school and on the SAT and stuff I got 50% extended time and I got to take the test in a separate room. Also, I got deadlines pushed back for my written assignments if I needed them.

Therapist: Were those things helpful?

Client: Yes! Oh, well, actually yes and no, I'd say. The extra time on tests was helpful because then I didn't stress out as much and I could be less distracted and actually think straight. But I don't think the separate room helped too much and sometimes it was, like, TOO quiet, you know?

Therapist: Ahh, I see! That makes sense. I've heard from some of my clients with ADHD that total silence is almost worse than a noisy room. And what about the deadline extensions?

Client: I mean, it probably helped my grades because I didn't get dinged for late work but it also meant that I just procrastinated longer sometimes, actually, and dragged out the stress even more.

Therapist: Okay, so it sounds like the extended time on tests did really help you "show what you know" but the separate room wasn't that helpful. And the flexible deadlines maybe helped your grade but didn't really help your learning or your ability to show what you know as much.

Client: Yeah, that's fair.

Therapist: So the extended time is a really good example of something that might really be helping you **access** the test in a way that provides a level playing field for you despite your ADHD, just like we talked about earlier. On the other hand, maybe a quiet room and flexible deadlines aren't really a good accommodation for your ADHD. Have you used any of these accommodations in college?

Client: Sort of. My mom really pushed me to register for them first semester freshman year but then I really didn't use them. I felt like I didn't want to bother my professors about it. And, I didn't like sitting in a separate little room by myself.

Therapist: I see. Do you think that the extended time accommodation by itself might be helpful now? Is that something that it might be worth learning more about?

Client: Yeah, maybe. I can see what I need to do to get that started again.

Therapist: Okay, cool. Are there any other areas academically that you feel like you're struggling with? Maybe things that we haven't really been able to address through the organization and study skills we've been working on? Any classes you're really struggling with right now, for example?

Client:	Ugh. YES. Things are going okay in most of my classes, but my stats class is killing me and it's only the third week of the semester. I've been to office hours with my professor, but I can only go once a week for 30 minutes because of my work schedule. I'm kind of worried I'm falling behind already.
Therapist:	Huh, that's stressful. I wonder if the Academic Skills Center has tutors for that class.
Client:	Wait, what?
Therapist:	Yeah, I've heard a lot of students struggle with their intro stats class so I know that Academic Skills has group tutoring for that class almost every semester. And, if there's no tutoring available for that specific class, you can request an individual tutor.
Client:	That's news to me. I honestly forgot that place existed.
Therapist:	Oh yeah, they're great! Sounds like making an appointment there would be a good homework assignment along with making one for Disability Services to talk about a testing accommodation. If so, let's look at how you book the appointments and what kind of paperwork you need before we wrap up today.

Plan Out Steps to Access Accommodations and Services

Collaboratively list out the steps the student will need to complete to request and arrange accommodations or other academic support services at their institution.

For disability accommodation requests, these steps will typically include:

1 Contact the campus Disability Services office or other responsible person to begin the process.
2 Gather existing documentation (e.g., testing records, assessment reports, high school IEP).
3 Attend the consultation ready to discuss primary difficulties with access and what you believe may be helpful accommodations.
4 Obtain additional disability documentation as needed.
5 Receive the disability accommodation notice (DAN) or letter of accommodation (LOA) and distribute to professors along with a request to meet to make arrangements for the accommodation. (Note: At some schools, the Disability Services office will handle distribution).
6 Meet with each professor to arrange how the accommodation will be provided – for example, will you take your tests at a campus testing center? Or will you arrive early to get started?
7 Maintain contact with the disability services provider if you have trouble getting your accommodations.

Note that the nature of these steps, particularly 5 and 6, will differ from school to school. For instance, at some institutions the campus Disability Services office will automatically distribute the DAN (LOA) to a student's professors when they are officially enrolled. In some instances, professors are then required to acknowledge receipt and also that they have read the letter. In all instances, students receiving disability services should check in with their instructors to make sure they are aware of their needs and also to ensure that they agree on how the approved accommodations will work.

For academic skills providers outside of disability services (e.g., university's Learning or Academic Skills Center), work with the student to identify the procedure for setting up an initial consultation, including where the office is physically located and how to arrange an appointment. Finally, encourage the student to add the steps of these plans to their task list and help them identify a day and time in their schedule to complete the first step.

Accommodations on High-stakes Tests

Students pursuing educational or career paths where high-stakes testing is required should be aware that the documentation standards for testing accommodations on these exams, such as the MCAT, LSAT, and GRE, may be more rigorous than for academic accommodations in college. For example, evaluators may need to be highly qualified in their field, the evidence presented may need to document not just a diagnosis but support the presence of disability (impairment in a major life activity compared to most people in the population) and the need for the specific accommodation to mitigate the effects of that disability. For example, an IEP from high school or a primary care doctor's note stating that a student has ADHD will likely not be sufficient for certain exams. Even a detailed report that addresses the ADHD diagnosis but *not* its effects on test-taking (e.g., reading speed) might not be enough to qualify a student for extended time on a test like the MCAT.

In addition, evaluations must typically be recent – for example, within the past three years. Students interested in receiving testing accommodations on these exams should determine the documentation requirements well ahead of when they plan to take the test so that they can obtain the needed documentation and submit their request for accommodations in sufficient time for their application to be evaluated.

Discuss Homework and Set the Next Meeting

Review the client's next steps for academic skills practice using the handout. Review any steps they identified for pursuing disability accommodations and other academic support on campus, make sure that they have put these steps on their calendar and task list. Finally, schedule the next session.

Note

1 These are very commonly requested accommodations; however, note that there is weak to no research support for extended time or any other accommodation as specifically "leveling the playing field" for students with ADHD (Lewandowski et al., 2013; Miller et al., 2015; Weis & Beauchemin, 2020).

References

Gordon, M., Lewandowski, L., & Lovett, B.J. (2015). Assessment and management of ADHD in educational and workplace settings in the context of ADA accommodations. In R.A. Barkley (Ed.), *Attention-deficit/hyperactivity disorder: A handbook for diagnosis and treatment* (fourth edition, pp. 774–794). Guilford Press.

Lewandowski, L., Gathje, R.A., Lovett, B.J., & Gordon, M. (2013). Test-taking skills in college students with and without ADHD. *Journal of Psychoeducational Assessment, 31*(1), 41–52. 10.1177/0734282912446304

Miller, L.A., Lewandowski, L.J., & Antshel, K.M. (2015). Effects of extended time for college students with and without ADHD. *Journal of Attention Disorders, 19*(8), 678–686. 10.1177/1087054713483308

Weis, R., & Beauchemin, E.L. (2020). Are separate room test accommodations effective for college students with disabilities? *Assessment & Evaluation in Higher Education, 45*(5), 794–809. 10.1080/02602938.2019.1702922

Skill 3: Thinking and Responding Differently

(~4 sessions)

Corresponds to Skillset 3 of the *Thriving in College* Student Workbook

Background for the Therapist

Although ADHD is a neurodevelopmental disorder and is not *caused by* a client's patterns of thinking, the cognitive lens through which a client with ADHD sees the world can contribute to the impairment that results from ADHD symptoms. Therefore, teaching clients to become more aware of their thoughts and to decouple those thoughts from problematic responses is a key strategy in many cognitive-behavioral approaches to adult ADHD (Safren et al., 2017).

The Cognitive Model of ADHD

As discussed in other sections of this manual, ADHD is a disorder of executive functioning that directly impacts a client's capacity to accomplish goals over time. This means that many people with ADHD, particularly when it is untreated, may fail to live up to what they or others perceive as "their potential." In addition, the impulsivity and emotional dysregulation associated with the disorder can cause damage to personal relationships and a higher-than-average rate of negative feedback and rejection from others. As such, by adulthood, people with ADHD have likely endured high rates of failure experiences that can lead to rigid internalized concepts, or *schemas*, about their capabilities and future potential. Ramsay (2020) recently proposed that impaired *self-regulatory efficacy* – or lack of belief in one's own ability to self-regulate – is the core cognitive theme in adult ADHD and that *self-mistrust* is a key schema. Given their life experience with self-regulation failure, adults with ADHD may assume that they will *never* be able to consistently achieve their goals, and that a future of letting down themselves and others is inevitable.

Thus, negative thinking in adults with ADHD not only *feels* bad, but it likely contributes to the very self-regulation failures that led to negative thinking in the first place. In particular, a pattern of negative thinking may contribute to avoidance and procrastination for people with ADHD (Ramsay, 2002; Safren et al., 2004). After all, if self-regulation failure seems inevitable, this leaves little motivation to persist in trying. As a group, adults with ADHD

DOI: 10.4324/9781003149590-13

report higher levels of the kinds of *negative automatic thoughts* often seen in depression and anxiety disorders (Mitchell et al., 2013), which are associated with avoidance behaviors and depression symptoms (Knouse et al., 2013). Negative thinking may be one process that contributes to the increased risk for depression and even suicidal behavior in this population (Eddy et al., 2018). To illustrate the potential role of negative automatic thoughts in avoidance, an adult with ADHD might be presented with the idea of trying to use a new calendar system and have the negative automatic thought, "I've tried that a thousand times. It's not going to work for me," which, unsurprisingly, might result in feeling demoralized and disengaging from this possibly-useful skill.

For adults with ADHD, problematic thoughts are not always negative in "flavor." Earlier in the history of the application of CBT to adult ADHD, clinicians began to recognize that these clients also seem to exhibit problematic *positive* automatic thoughts – that is, thoughts with optimistic, "rose-colored" content that contribute to failure to employ needed self-regulation skills (Mitchell et al., 2008; Ramsay & Rostain, 2008; Sprich et al., 2010). For ex-ample, clients might be confronted with an important task and think, "I've got plenty of time to work on that tomorrow," or, "I'll feel ready to do that later," and then fail to engage with the task, putting it off until consequences are dire and anxiety is overwhelming. Such thinking can often be related to client dif-ficulties in accurately judging and using time. These "positive" but problematic thoughts may also temporarily soothe negative emotions such as anxiety or discomfort, leading to negative reinforcement of such patterns of thinking, despite maladaptive avoidance behavior that follows (Knouse & Mitchell, 2015). For example, if a student has a class project due in a few weeks and they misjudge how much time is needed for the project due to overly optimistic thinking, they might end up submitting a lower quality project and experien-cing a much higher level of stress than necessary to complete the project on time. Given preliminary evidence that these avoidance-related thoughts occur more frequently for adults with ADHD (Knouse et al., 2019), the sessions that follow also prompt clients to become aware of these thinking patterns and respond to them with engagement with self-regulation rather than avoidance.

Strategies in this Skillset

The overarching goal of this set of skills is to teach clients how to practice and maintain new, adaptive cognitive and behavioral responses in the presence of challenging and problematic thoughts and feelings. First, clients will practice **mindfulness techniques** and then learn to **self-observe in emotionally challenging situations**. Next, they will learn to engage in **self-monitoring of thoughts, feelings, and behavior** in daily life and conduct **functional assessment** of the relations among these experiences. Next, clients will develop and practice **alternative cognitive and behavioral responses** to these patterns in daily life. Finally, you will guide clients in applying these skills to the most difficult situations – those that require clients to **manage impulsivity and regulate emotions**.

Therapists familiar with cognitive-behavioral therapy for depression and anxiety disorders will, no doubt, be well acquainted with all of the skills in this section. While these skills do not form the core of CBT for ADHD, they are often crucial to successful *implementation* of self-regulation skills in daily life (Knouse, 2015; Ramsay, 2016). Furthermore, given the high rates of comorbid mood and anxiety symptoms and disorders experienced by adults with ADHD (Kessler et al., 2006), these skills may be useful in addressing these associated problems.

Experienced therapists may note that we take the somewhat unusual approach of teaching mindfulness skills as a precursor to training in formal self-monitoring of thoughts, feelings and behaviors. We believe that the first crucial strategy in this set of skills is to teach adults with ADHD **to become aware of the relation among problematic thoughts, feelings, and avoidance behaviors.** We assume that awareness is a necessary condition for being able to practice new responses to these patterns when they occur in daily life. Given the cardinal ADHD symptoms of inattention and impulsivity, many adults with ADHD may have difficulty self-observing their own responses and therefore beginning cognitive work with mindfulness skills may enhance their ability to self-monitor. Therapists will also note that our treatment does not require clients to commit to a long-term mindfulness practice – for example, mindfulness meditation – that is separate from their daily life experiences. Although clients are invited to develop such a practice and there is growing evidence that it could be beneficial, our approach emphasizes the application of mindfulness in daily life.

This set of skills concludes with the specific application of cognitive and behavioral strategies to situations in which the client experiences strong emotions that contribute to problematic impulsivity. ADHD has been associated with emotional dysregulation and, in particular, difficulties with impulsive responding in the presence of strong negative emotions such as frustration (Barkley, 2010). Emotional impulsivity has been associated with impairments in work, education, driving, and financial outcomes among adults whose ADHD persisted from childhood (Barkley & Fischer, 2010). Impulsive behavior in the presence of strong negative emotion – in other words, the tendency to act impulsively when distressed – is referred to as **negative urgency** (Cyders & Smith, 2008). Importantly, negative urgency has been shown to partially explain the relation between ADHD and risk for substance abuse in adults (Egan et al., 2017; Pedersen et al., 2016, 2019; Roberts et al., 2014). Impulsivity may also increase in the presence of positive emotions such as excitement. **Positive urgency** describes this tendency to act impulsively in the presence of strong positive affect (Cyders & Smith, 2008). In adulthood, positive urgency has also been associated with increased risk for alcohol problems (Pedersen et al., 2016, 2019) and other substance use for people with ADHD, although less robustly than negative urgency (Egan et al., 2017). Given the important relations between regulation of negative and positive emotions and risk for impulsive behavior, our approach to helping clients reduce impulsivity focuses on applying skills to respond differently in the presence of strong emotions. Inspired by the approach of Deffenbacher and McKay (2000) to reducing angry responding, our approach engages clients in ***impulsivity inoculation*** exercises in which the client will use imaginal exposure and covert rehearsal to practice their new responses to the situations and emotions that lead to impulsive responding.

Student Workbook

If you are using the *Thriving in College* student workbook, you will find that Skillset 3 on *Thinking and Doing Differently* corresponds to the material in this section. The following chart provides more information on which individual modules in the workbook correspond to each session in this section.

Therapist Guide Session	*Workbook Modules*
1	3.0 Why it Matters, Pre-Assessment, & Roadmap
	3.1 Becoming Aware Through Mindfulness
2	3.2 Notice Your Patterns
3	3.3 Practice New Responses I
4	3.4 Practice New Responses II: Hot Thoughts and Impulsivity

References

Barkley, R.A. (2010). Deficient emotional self-regulation is a core component of ADHD. *Journal of ADHD and Related Disorders, 1*(2), 5–37.

Barkley, R.A., & Fischer, M. (2010). The unique contribution of emotional impulsiveness to impairment in major life activities in hyperactive children as adults. *Journal of the American Academy of Child & Adolescent Psychiatry, 49*(5), 503–513. 10.1016/j.jaac. 2010.01.019

Beck, J.S. (2011). *Cognitive behavior therapy: Basics and beyond* (Second Edition). Guilford Press.

Cyders, M.A., & Smith, G.T. (2008). Emotion-based dispositions to rash action: Positive and negative urgency. *Psychological Bulletin, 134*(6), 807–828. 10.1037/a0013341

Deffenbacher, J.L., & McKay, M. (2000). *Overcoming situational and general anger: A Protocol for the treatment of anger based on relaxation, cognitive restructuring, and coping Skills.* New Harbinger.

Eddy, L.D., Dvorsky, M.R., Molitor, S.J., Bourchtein, E., Smith, Z., Oddo, L.E., Eadeh, H.-M., & Langberg, J.M. (2018). Longitudinal evaluation of the cognitive-behavioral model of ADHD in a sample of college students With ADHD. *Journal of Attention Disorders, 22*(4), 323–333. 10.1177/1087054715616184

Egan, T.E., Dawson, A.E., & Wymbs, B.T. (2017). Substance use in undergraduate students with histories of attention-deficit/hyperactivity disorder (ADHD): The role of impulsivity. *Substance Use & Misuse, 52*(10), 1375–1386. 10.1080/10826084.2017. 1281309

Kessler, R.C., Adler, L., Barkley, R.A., Biederman, J., Conners, C.K., Demler, O. et al. (2006). The prevalence and correlates of adult ADHD in the United States: Results from the National Comorbidity Survey Replication. *American Journal of Psychiatry, 163*(4), 716–723. 10.1176/appi.ajp.163.4.716

Knouse, L.E. (2015). Treatment of adults with ADHD: Cognitive-behavioral therapies for ADHD. In R.A. Barkley (Ed.), *Attention-Deficit Hyperactivity Disorder: A Handbook for Diagnosis and Treatment* (4th ed., pp. 757–773). Guilford Press.

Knouse, L.E., & Mitchell, J.T. (2015). Incautiously optimistic: Positively valenced cognitive avoidance in adult adhd. *Cognitive and Behavioral Practice, 22*(2), 192–202. 10.1016/ j.cbpra.2014.06.003

Knouse, L.E., Mitchell, J.T., Kimbrel, N.A., & Anastopoulos, A.D. (2019). Development and evaluation of the ADHD cognitions scale for adults. *Journal of Attention Disorders, 23*(10), 1090–1100. 10.1177/1087054717707580

Knouse, L.E., Zvorsky, I., & Safren, S.A. (2013). Depression in adults with attention-deficit/hyperactivity disorder (ADHD): The mediating role of cognitive-behavioral factors. *Cognitive Therapy and Research, 37*(6), 1220–1232. 10.1007/s10608-013-9569-5

Mitchell, J.T., Benson, J.W., Knouse, L.E., Kimbrel, N.A., & Anastopoulos, A.D. (2013). Are negative automatic thoughts associated with ADHD in adulthood? *Cognitive Therapy and Research, 37*(4), 851–859. 10.1007/s10608-013-9525-4

Mitchell, J.T., Nelson-Gray, R.O., & Anastopoulos, A.D. (2008). Adapting an emerging empirically supported cognitive-behavioral therapy for adults with ADHD and comorbid complications: An example of two case studies. *Clinical Case Studies, 7*, 423–448.

Pedersen, S.L., King, K.M., Louie, K.A., Fournier, J.C., & Molina, B.S.G. (2019). Momentary fluctuations in impulsivity domains: Associations with a history of childhood ADHD, heavy alcohol use, and alcohol problems. *Drug and Alcohol Dependence, 205*, 107683. 10.1016/j.drugalcdep.2019.107683

Pedersen, S.L., Walther, C.A.P., Harty, S.C., Gnagy, E.M., Pelham, W.E., & Molina, B.S.G. (2016). The indirect effects of childhood attention deficit hyperactivity disorder on alcohol problems in adulthood through unique facets of impulsivity. *Addiction, 111*(9), 1582–1589. 10.1111/add.13398

Ramsay, J.R. (2002). A cognitive therapy approach for treating chronic procrastination and avoidance: Behavioral activation interventions. *Journal of Group Psychotherapy, Psychodrama & Sociometry (15453855), 55*(2/3), 79–92. 10.3200/ JGPP.55.2.79-92

Ramsay, J.R. (2016). Turning intentions into actions": CBT for adult adhd focused on implementation. *Clinical Case Studies, 15*(3), 179–197. 10.1177/1534650115611483

Ramsay, J.R. (2020). *Rethinking adult ADHD: Helping clients turn intentions into actions.* American Psychological Association.

Ramsay, J.R., & Rostain, A. (2008). *Cognitive-behavioral therapy for adult ADHD: An integrative psychosocial and medical approach.* Routledge/Taylor & Francis Group.

Roberts, W., Peters, J.R., Adams, Z.W., Lynam, D.R., & Milich, R. (2014). Identifying the facets of impulsivity that explain the relation between ADHD symptoms and substance use in a nonclinical sample. *Addictive Behaviors, 39*(8), 1272–1277. 10.1016/j.addbeh.2014.04.005

Safren, S.A., Sprich, S., Perlman, C.A., & Otto, M.W. (2017). *Mastering your adult ADHD: A cognitive behavioral treatment program, therapist guide* (2nd ed.). Oxford University Press.

Safren, S., Sprich, S., Chulvick, S., & Otto, M.W. (2004). Psychosocial treatments for adults with attention-deficit/hyperactivity disorder. *Psychiatric Clinics of North America, 27*(2), 349–360. 10.1016/S0193-953X(03)00089-3

Sprich, S., Knouse, L.E., Cooper-Vince, C., Burbridge, J., & Safren, S.A. (2010). Description and demonstration of CBT for ADHD in adults. *Cognitive and Behavioral Practice, 17*(1), 9–15. 10.1016/j.cbpra.2009.09.002

Session 1: Being Mindful

Corresponds to Module 3.1 in the *Thriving in College* Student Workbook

Session Outline

1 Check-in with client(s)
2 Set agenda
3 Discuss the concept of mindfulness and how ADHD makes this hard
4 Complete mindfulness self-assessment
5 Discuss self-monitoring
6 Complete self-monitoring exercise
7 Discuss mindfulness practice
8 Complete mindfulness exercise
9 Discuss other mindful activities
10 Discuss homework
11 Schedule the next session

Session Organization

Administration Format

Session 1 can be administered in a group or individual format. A group session may be optimal in that the presence of others can evoke sensations and thoughts and feelings that are useful fodder for self-monitoring and mindfulness practice. Sharing and hearing prior experiences with meditation, yoga, or other similar activities can also be helpful. However, the session can also be efficiently and effectively employed for an individual client, if a group format is not practical.

Materials Needed

The therapist should ready for demonstration or discussion two or three iOS and/or Android applications that can be used for meditation, yoga, or other mindful activities that clients can explore further on their own.

DOI: 10.4324/9781003149590-14

- A whiteboard, flipchart, or a projected digital document is recommended to capture group ideas and/or present material, as well as a list of "take home messages" regarding the session's content as well as instructions/goals for at-home work prior to the next session.
- Finally, bring (or distribute ahead of time) worksheets (see examples below) that facilitate self-monitoring, for use in session and between sessions.

As always, therapists are reminded to instruct clients ahead of the session to bring a notebook or device on which they can take notes.

Session Content

Check-in with Client(s)

It is unlikely that this will be the first technique or content-heavy session that a client has done with you. Check-in time can be used to solicit brief discussion, or simply to see how things are going and build rapport. In the event that this session is the first meeting with clients, check-in might focus more on feelings and expectations about therapy. In any event, aim for this to be brief (< 5 minutes), encouraging for any additional discussion of this sort to be postponed until after the session content is completed. See therapist-client check-in dialogue example in Skill 1: Session 1 as a model for this interaction, if needed. We also recommend having your client complete the *Progress Tracker* (see Appendix B), and briefly touching base on any declines or improvements in school functioning.

Set Agenda

Introduce the agenda for this session to the client (see Session Outline). It may be helpful to have a visual aid to refer to, such as a flip chart or projected PowerPoint slide or printed handout. At this time it might also be helpful to remind clients to write notes regarding important points in a therapy notebook. Setting the agenda should be speedily completed (< 2 minutes). See therapist-client agenda-setting dialogue example in Skill 1: Session 1 as a model, if needed.

Discuss the Concept of Mindfulness and How ADHD Can Make It Hard

As discussed, ADHD is a disorder that is at least partly defined by inattention and distraction. Distraction plays out for people with ADHD all the time in their lives, down to their moment-to-moment activity. People with ADHD often lament getting off track from what they want to be doing and *not even noticing* that they are off track until much later, often to the point where they don't finish the task they intended to. Besides getting distracted by competing activities (e.g., playing a video game instead of doing homework), students with ADHD can also get derailed by anxious, dysphoric, or just daydreamy thoughts. Simply thinking in these divergent ways can be like a mental whirlpool; it is hard to extract oneself from it, and it overwhelms more adaptive possibilities.

Being in these kinds of behavioral or cognitive states can feel a bit like being on "automatic pilot" (Zylowska, 2012). A common experience that illustrates this automatic pilot occurs when driving on the highway. Drivers can experience getting into a kind of mental zone where they become less immediately aware of the cars around them, of their own actions, of time and distance going by. This, in several ways, is very different from the state of mindfulness, which has been shown to be a promising cognitive tool for people with ADHD (Mitchell et al., 2017). Being mindful involves meta-awareness, or, in other words, the ability to observe your thoughts, feelings, and behaviors as they are happening. Mindfulness can be described as a personal, cognitive orientation involving two aspects:

- Consistent yet flexible **attention to what is happening in the present moment** – this can include one's behaviors, thoughts, or feelings, or things occurring around oneself
- Maintaining a **nonjudgmental attitude** toward one's observations of what is happening – this means being curious, open, and accepting about one's experiences

Mindfulness, as a practice, is popularly linked to meditation (e.g., Zen Buddhism), so you might want to check in with clients about any experience they have had in the past with this type of activity. Cultivating one's mindfulness can begin with simple exercises (e.g., paying attention to one's breath). Mindfulness often involves conscious awareness of all five of our senses in our current experience, many of which may be automatically neglected otherwise. One exercise involving awareness of senses is mindful eating (e.g., a grape, a cup of tea); a client may be able to reflect on how sight, sound, and tactile sensations might be commonly ignored in this activity. In general, being fully mindful allows one to *notice* what one is doing in any given moment – whether it is having a particular sensation or thought, engaging in a behavior, or having a feeling) – and being able to *selectively attend* to that current activity or *flexibly shift attention* to something else, and keep one's attention there. These are things that people with ADHD tend to have difficulty with, and so the practice of mindfulness can help decrease distraction and procrastination, while also helping to regulate negative emotions like frustration or anxiety. Further, mindful awareness of thoughts, feelings, and actions can give clients a chance to choose different responses in situations that are typically problematic. Talking with your client(s) about the potential benefits of mindfulness could help build motivation to complete at-home exercises and strengthen their mindfulness skills (see Dialogue 1 for an example).

Dialogue 1

Therapist:	*I'd like to talk with you all a little bit about mindfulness, which is the main strategy we are going to be working on today. This is something that has ties to traditional meditation practices. I'm curious as to whether any of you have ever tried meditation before?*
Client (one of several in the group):	*Well, yeah, I think so … I've done some yoga classes, and I think that in the quiet moments between or after the physical stretching the instructor has had us do this.*
Therapist:	*OK, great! So tell us what you remember about that.*
Client:	*I remember that the instructor had us focus on our breathing, and also on how different parts of our bodies felt. I remember that I noticed things that I never have before, and also being really relaxed.*
Therapist:	*So it sounds like you directed your focus to different sorts of things, and also that you noticed things that you hadn't before. I'm also hearing that you thought it was a neat experience.*
Client:	*Totally. I remember feeling like my mind was expanded, but at the same time that I could stay focused on something in a relaxed sort of way.*
Therapist:	*That's great, it is actually very much what we want to cultivate as a skill in this group! It doesn't have to be something that someone does just during yoga, or in some other class. Mindfulness is a practice that can be used just about anywhere, and it involves consistent attention to your current experience. What feelings and sensations you have, what your thoughts are, what's happening around you. Being mindful in your everyday life is a good technique to "catch" when you are starting to do something that's different from what you wanted to, and to redirect your focus back.*
Client (another in the group):	*I have done some yoga, too, and I remember the yoga instructor saying that if something distracted me that was OK, that I could just bring my attention back to my breath or legs or whatever. That felt good.*
Therapist:	*Right! So the idea here really is when you notice lots of things, even things that are away from where you want your attention to be, you shouldn't be harsh with yourself. It isn't a reason to negatively judge yourself. It's actually kind of natural to shift attention. And noticing that can be good … "hey, there's this thing that's happening …"*

	because if it's important, you can shift your focus. But if it's not critical, you can kind of acknowledge it, and let it go ... and just come back to what you want to have your attention on.
Client:	*OK, yeah.*
Therapist:	*So, for all of you, how would it feel to be able to use this kind of thinking anywhere, not just in yoga?*
Client (a third in the group):	*I personally think it would be cool. I might be able to be more focused on what I want, and also less upset and down on myself if I notice myself going off the tracks.*
Therapist:	*You know, I think it would be cool too. I think you really might like this. Shall we give this a try?*
Clients:	*Yeah, let's do it.*

Complete Mindfulness Self-assessment

At this point in the session, it is useful to do a mindfulness check-in with the client to see where they are at the present moment. The Toronto Mindfulness Scale (Lau et al., 2006) is a validated measure that taps the two principal aspects of mindfulness: "decentering" and "curiosity." Appendix B presents two versions of the scale. The first, which you should use here, is a measure of how the person *generally* acts on a continuum from un-mindful to very mindful (the second version assesses *state* mindfulness and might be a good tool to use in session to demonstrate change following mindful practice). Have the client complete the general (i.e., "trait") version of the scale and score using the instructions on the form. You might discuss the results but keep it brief. The purpose of completing the assessment is to help the client to become aware of their own general orientation and to help them see if mindfulness practice changes this (i.e., reassessing after mindful practice has been done for a few weeks, either right after using the state version, or as a general assessment, using the trait version).

Discuss Self-monitoring

Self-monitoring can be likened to the first principle of mindfulness that you will introduce to the client. It is all about *awareness* of one's feelings, thoughts, and behaviors. Discuss with the client how remaining aware seems like a simple thing but how we are programmed to not self-monitor in many different situations. The concept of "ballistic" movements may be helpful here; this aspect of human behavior encapsulates complex behaviors that are in a sense programmed, made up of many smaller behavioral steps. So, as an example, we often fail to self-monitor when we brush our teeth, when we get dressed in the morning, when we start a car. We have done these things so many times that our brain channels attention to other things besides the behaviors that make up these actions. So, while you are brushing your teeth, you think about the things that you need to do that morning. While you are starting the car, you may be most aware of how cold it is outside. There are other routines that become similarly automatic, such as reciting *The Pledge of Allegiance* for American schoolchildren. While this process creates efficiencies in our lives where we can do two or more things at once, at the same time it is a failure of self-monitoring.

Unfortunately, self-monitoring "efficiency" is not always a positive thing. For example, when we are feeling anxious, we often fail to notice what we are actually thinking (e.g., "I really hope this person won't think I'm a freak!") and how we are behaving (e.g., fiddling with the drawstrings on my hoodie). Clients with ADHD may identify with this example: when one gets distracted from a task (e.g., studying) and begins doing something else (e.g., gaming), both the fact that the new activity is being done and that the prior intention to finish the task has been abandoned go virtually unnoticed. Talk with the client about these self-monitoring failures and others, including the idea that there is always *something* that is occurring inside or around us that goes unnoticed that we could draw our awareness to. Discuss how the client may have noticed failures of self-monitoring being problematic and introduce the idea that being able to se-lectively activate self-monitoring in their daily life could be beneficial to staying on track, avoiding spiraling anxiety or dysphoria, and generally making better choices.

Complete Self-monitoring Exercise

While the therapy session may not be the most complex situation in which the client could engage in self-monitoring, it still provides an opportunity to demonstrate the basic principles. You are going to assign self-monitoring homework (see below), so the goal of this practice is just to get the hang of using the self-monitoring form. Take a few minutes to work through the self-monitoring form found in Appendix A, encouraging the client to move through awareness and monitoring of their feelings, thoughts, behaviors, and sensations of events in the environment around them.

Discuss Mindfulness Practice

Like self-monitoring, mindfulness, which not only encompasses awareness but also *selective* attention and the nonjudgmental and accepting psychological posture, is something that can be cultivated through intentional practice. One's ability to be mindful, like one's ability to lift weights, for example, is something that can be improved over time through effortful repetition. There are two ways that mindfulness can be practiced in the client's life, both of which you want to encourage given the possible benefits of being able to notice distraction or upset, being able to recognize what is happening that may influence these states, and then being able to selectively change one's focus to be better adapted in the moment. Both *formal* and *informal* mindfulness practice are important (Zylowska, 2012). Continuing the analogy of building muscle, formal practice is like having a regular gym routine to build strength and endurance. The type of exercise that you will do with the client could be done daily at a scheduled time and chosen place to facilitate formal practice. Informal practice is like taking advantage of opportunities in your daily life that might build more fitness, such as walking up two flights of stairs instead of taking the elevator. Informal mindfulness can be practiced in any quiet or even chaotic moment. For instance, while riding a bus, the client could mindfully attend to their breath, their thoughts, their sensations, the events in the environment around them, any feelings they are experiencing, and then return their awareness back to their breath, and continue this as a cycle. Discuss these concepts with the client, encouraging them to see that mindfulness practice might not take much time, can easily fit into their everyday lives, and may provide attentional and emotional benefits.

Complete Mindfulness Exercise

This mindful breathing exercise is one that will require you to read a script verbatim to the client (see Box 1, following page). It should take approximately 15 minutes to complete this exercise and debrief with the client, checking in on their experiences, highlighting positive feelings they may have, and making suggestions about difficulties. Note that many people engaging in mindfulness will, at first, complain that their attention wanders or that they keep having thoughts or sensations or feelings that are distracting from the instruction to focus on one's breath. Try to encourage the client by saying that such experiences during mindfulness practice are typical and an illustration of mindfulness itself: noticing things in the internal and external environment and then bringing attention back to the intended focus. This is flexing a mental muscle that is particularly useful for college students with ADHD; note that this becomes easier and second nature with practice.

Discuss Other Mindful Activities

There are several other, simple, intentional mindfulness activities that your client(s) can use in daily life to practice the central aspects of mindfulness, maintaining their attention on what is happening in the present moment and adopting the nonjudgmental attitude toward what they perceive to be happening. We have included a few of these in Box 2, along with brief instructions on how they could be carried out. We suggest discussing these with

Box 1   Mindful Breathing Exercise

The first thing for you to do is to get yourself into a comfortable position. A lot of people find that sitting in a supportive chair, one that's not too cushy, is best, keeping both feet on the ground, and letting their arms either rest on the arms of the chair (if there are any) or just hang down naturally, with their hands in their lap. Some people, when they are at home, will try this lying down, on a couch or bed. This is OK as long as you are not very tired ... the rhythmic nature of this exercise can naturally relax you and you may fall asleep, so again, it's good to sit upright, in a comfortable position.

OK, now, close your eyes. This will help you focus, which is important as you practice this exercise. Once you've done this, direct your attention to your breath. This is about noticing what is always there with us, but that which we seldom attend to.

Breathe in through your nose, and out through your mouth. Take deep breaths, filling your lungs each time so that your belly expands when you inhale fully. Focus on breathing deeper and slower than usual. Hold your breath for two or three seconds after you fill your lungs, and then exhale through your mouth, slowly, completely. Empty your lungs every time you exhale. As you are doing this, if you find your mind wandering to other things, thoughts, feelings, sensations, just notice what is happening. Tell yourself that is OK, it is natural ... accept it ... but then, gently, redirect your attention to your breathing. Continue with this pattern of breathing for a minute or so. Just breathe deeply, and keep drawing your attention back to your breath, if it wanders.

Now, as you continue to breathe deeply, notice how it feels to breathe in. Focus on the inhalations. Notice that the air that comes into your nostrils may feel cool. What noise do you make when you do this? Notice what it feels like for your chest to expand, for your lungs to fill. Feel the tension, the fullness, as you hold your deep breath, before you exhale. Again, your attention may naturally go to something else ... acknowledge to yourself when this happens, and then peacefully and without judgment bring your attention back to your breath. Do this for a minute or so.

Next, focus on what it is like when you exhale. Notice how the breath that leaves your mouth is now warmer than when it came in. Feel your lungs release the air, completely. Notice how your stomach, and your chest, deflates or gets smaller. Does it feel relaxing to let the air go completely? Do you notice the urge, the insistence, of your body, before you take the next breath? Continue with this for another minute, and if you find yourself thinking about something else, gently bring your focus back to your breath.

Continue breathing for another minute, noticing all the sensations, the feelings, of deep breathing.

Now, I want you to continue breathing as you have been, but I want you to consciously let your attention open more widely. Things will begin to come to your awareness, naturally ... and then you may want to direct yourself to notice certain things. Are there any sounds in the room, or the building, that you are in right now? (Pause.) *If there are sounds that are identifiable, what are they? If there are sounds that are vague, what do you think they could be?* (Pause.) *How does your body feel right now? (Pause.) What about specific parts of your body? Your hands? Your legs? Your arms? Your back? Your shoulders? Your head? (Pause.) What does the air around you feel like? Are there any smells? Do you notice a draft, or is it warm, or cold? (Pause.) Now, let go of these physical sensations … and let whatever thoughts may come, come. Notice these. Acknowledge them. Then try to let each go … see what comes next. You might imagine each thought floating away, as if it were a leaf floating downstream, and then the next thought comes, as if you notice a new leaf, floating into your sight. (Pause.) Maybe, as you are doing this, a feeling may begin. What is that feeling? Be specific. How strongly are you feeling that feeling? Stay with it. Acknowledge that the feeling is there. Now, just as you did with your thoughts, try to let that feeling go … and see what comes next … . (Pause.)*

Continue keeping your mind and your focus open … let there be a curiosity there … what will come next? See what that is, whatever it is … and then, again, shift your awareness away, and let what comes next, come. (Two minute pause.)

Now, I would like you to gently, slowly, redirect your focus intentionally to your breath. Focus on the sensations of your deep breathing. Notice the tension, then the relaxation. The air coming all the way into your belly, and then whooshing out through your mouth. Continue focusing on these and the other sensations of your breath, and if your mind wanders, that's OK, notice that, then bring it back to center, to your breath. Continue to do this for another minute.

After this last minute has passed, you can slowly instruct the client(s) to open their eyes, to become aware of where they are again, and to let the intentional mindfulness go. In the debriefing, you can start by asking the client to simply talk about what they experienced. Reinforce or introduce that in the moment, any moment, we focus on only a limited number of things, and that there are others that are outside our awareness, until we mentally step back, and allow ourselves to notice them. After noticing these things, it is possible to stay with them, or to let them go, and redirect our attention to where we want it to be. This last aspect should be particularly emphasized for the client, as people with ADHD often have difficulty noticing that their attention has wandered when they are engaging in tasks or are in conversations or other activities, and the practice of mindfulness can build important adaptive skills that can generalize to everyday life.

the client and deploying them as they seem desired. If mindfulness becomes a useful practice and is adopted by your client, you might also try using one of these variant exercises in a future session to help them "mix it up." Further, there are many other resources that are available in print and online that clients can use to engage in more mindfulness, mediation, and other related techniques that can strengthen their mastery of this skill. See Box 2 for several options that

Box 2   Mindfulness activities and resources

Activities

Mindful eating: Take a grape (or raisin, or chocolate chip, or a berry) and focus on this with all of your senses, in turn. Take time to examine it, focusing on how it looks. As you do this, how does it feel in your hand? What about when you touch it with your fingertips? How does it smell? When you finally put it in your mouth, what does it taste like without chewing? How does it feel in your mouth? What about when you roll it around with your tongue? How are the tastes changing? Notice other things that may be happening in your body, like maybe saliva being released, or rumbling in your stomach. What happens on your first chew? What happens to the taste? Notice the texture of the food, too. Chew slowly, and notice these things. When the bite is fully chewed, swallow, and notice the feeling of swallowing, the taste that lingers in your mouth. How long does the taste stay there? Notice as it goes slowly away. During this process, if your attention wanders to thoughts, or feelings, or events around you, notice that, and nonjudgmentally turn your focus back to the morsel.

Mindful walking: It's nice to do this somewhere outside, in nature, but it can be done in an indoor space that's big enough to walk around unhindered, too. Start from a seated, relaxed position, noticing the sensations in your body, particularly those in your muscles. Take in how that feels, keeping your attention on your body. Notice your breathing. Can you feel your heart beating? Next, stand up, and notice how shifting your weight changes the sensations in your body. Where do you feel it most? What is it like? Next, begin to walk slowly. What are the physical sensations like? Do you sense your shifting balance, your muscles working? What changes are happening inside of you? How does the air feel? Different from sitting? As you walk, what do you hear around you? Are you making noise as you walk? Do you smell anything around you? Do you notice your breathing changing? How? What about your heart rate? Try changing your pace. Notice what changes as you do this. Keep mindfully noticing the sensations in your body, and continue this exercise for five minutes. During this process, if your attention wanders to thoughts, or feelings, or events around you, notice that, and nonjudgmentally turn your focus back to your walking

Books (may be available in audiobook or Kindle formats)
Zylowska, Lidia (2012). *The Mindfulness Prescription for Adult ADHD*. Trumpeter Books.
Kabat-Zinn (2016). *Mindfulness for Beginners*. Sounds True Publishing.

Shapiro, Shauna, & Siegel, Daniel (2020). *Good Morning, I Love You: Mindfulness and Self-Compassion Practices to Rewire Your Brain for Calm, Clarity, and Joy*. Sounds True Publishing.

Websites
Mindful: Happy Mind, Happy Life. www.mindful.org
Oxford Mindfulness Centre. Pay-per-course but also has free resources that are very helpful at https://www.oxfordmindfulness.org/learn-mindfulness/resources/
Tasting Mindfulness. Blog by Lynn Rossy, Ph.D., a health psychologist focusing on mindful eating, moving, and living. Lots of interesting content. https://www.lynnrossy.com/tasting-mindfulness/

Apps (Android/iOS)
Headspace
Mindfulness
Calm

Yoga
Many, many resources out there. University-based student recreation centers and other campus organizations undoubtedly offer yoga classes, including introductory ones. Many online yoga workouts are also available. If your client is interested in this more physical mindfulness activity, work with them to identify good starting options that are locally available.

were available at the time this manual was written. We strongly recommend, however, that you verify that they are currently available before passing them on to your client(s).

Discuss Homework and Schedule the Next Session

Suggested homework for clients after this session includes:

- Practice mindful breathing exercise 1x/daily.
- Choose and try at least one other mindfulness activity a few times in the next week.
- Before and after mindfulness exercises, complete the current-state version of the *Toronto Mindfulness scale* (see Appendix B), and record before and after scores for discussion at the next session (or for personal use, depending on client circumstance).
- Reflect on mindfulness practice in a daily journal, also for check-in at the next session and for personal insight.
- Complete a self-monitoring form at least three times in the next week.

References

Kabat-Zinn, J. (2016). *Mindfulness for beginners: Reclaiming the present moment and your life.* Sounds True.

Lau, M.A., Bishop, S.R., Segal, Z.V., Buis, T., Anderson, N.D., Carlson, L., Shapiro, S., Carmody, J., Abbey, S., & Devins, G. (2006). The Toronto Mindfulness Scale: Development and validation. *Journal of Clinical Psychology, 62*(12), 1445–1467. 10.1 002/jclp.20326

Mitchell, J.T., McIntyre, E.M., English, J.S., Dennis, M.F., Beckham, J.C., & Kollins, S.H. (2017). A pilot trial of mindfulness meditation training for ADHD in adulthood: Impact on core symptoms, executive functioning, and emotion dysregulation. *Journal of Attention Disorders, 21*(13), 1105–1120. 10.1177/1087054713513328

Shapiro, S., & Siegel, D. (2020). *Good morning, I love you: Mindfulness and self-compassion practices to rewire your brain for calm, clarity, and joy.* Sounds True.

Zylowska L. (2012). *The mindfulness prescription for adult ADHD: An 8-step program for strengthening attention, managing emotions, and achieving your goals.* Trumpeter.

Session 2: Noticing Your Patterns

Corresponds to Module 3.2 in the *Thriving in College* Student Workbook

Session Outline

1 Check-in with client(s)
2 Set agenda
3 Review homework from previous session
4 Discuss the cognitive model – relations between thoughts, feelings, and actions
5 Present the Daily Thought Record (DTR; self-monitoring version) with examples
6 Discuss self-monitoring with the DTR
7 Set homework
8 Schedule next session

Session Organization

Administration Format

Session 2 and Session 3 work in tandem to first **raise clients' awareness** of the relations among their thoughts, feelings, and behaviors and then to **begin to practice new cognitive and behavioral responses** in instances in which they are vulnerable to avoidant or otherwise problematic actions. Keep in mind that these are very challenging skills that, by themselves, are the key intervention strategies of many cognitive-behavioral treatments, such as CBT for depressive disorders (Beck, 2011). Two sessions spent on these skills should be considered the minimum duration. Many clients would benefit from more than two sessions to fully learn these skills and all clients will need support to continue practicing their new cognitive and behavioral responses throughout the remainder of the treatment and beyond. You should flexibly determine the amount of time spent on these skills based on your client's needs and preferences.

Materials Needed

Use a whiteboard, flipchart, or a projected/shared digital document to illustrate the cognitive model and work through client examples. You should also provide

DOI: 10.4324/9781003149590-15

clients access to paper or electronic handouts of Version 1 (self-monitoring version) of the Daily Thought Record (see Appendix A).

Session Content

Use this time to solicit brief discussion, or simply to see how things are going and build rapport. In the event that this session is the first meeting with clients, check-in might focus more on feelings and expectations about therapy. In any event, aim for this to be brief (< 5 minutes), encouraging for any additional discussion of this sort to be postponed until after the session content is completed. See therapist-client check-in dialogue example in Skill 1: Session 1 as a model for this interaction, if needed. We also recommend having your client complete the *Progress Tracker* (see Appendix B), and briefly touching base on any declines or improvements in school functioning.

Set Agenda

Introduce the agenda for this session to the client (see Session Outline). It may be helpful to have a visual aid to refer to, such as a flip chart or projected PowerPoint slide or printed handout. At this time, it might also be helpful to remind clients to write notes regarding important points in a therapy notebook. Setting the agenda should be speedily completed (< 2 minutes). See therapist-client agenda-setting dialogue example in Skill 1: Session 1 as a model, if needed.

Review Homework from Previous Session

Referring to your notes and the prior module completed, briefly remind the client what their homework assignment was and discuss successes and barriers to completion. See therapist-client agenda-setting dialogue example in Skill 1: Session 1 as a model, if needed.

Present the Cognitive Model of ADHD

Introduce and teach the cognitive model of ADHD using examples from the client's life (see Figure 1). A clear understanding of the model forms a foundation for using the Daily Thought Record (DTR) for self-monitoring, which will be part of clients' homework assignment for the next session.

ADHD itself is not caused by patterns of maladaptive thinking, yet living a lifetime with ADHD can contribute to thinking habits that can get in the way of clients using self-regulation skills. Teaching the client about the cognitive model of ADHD can help them begin to recognize the impact of maladaptive thinking patterns in their own lives (see Dialogue 1 for an example). This discussion can also serve to validate the client's experiences of the impact of ADHD on their self-concept and emotional well-being.

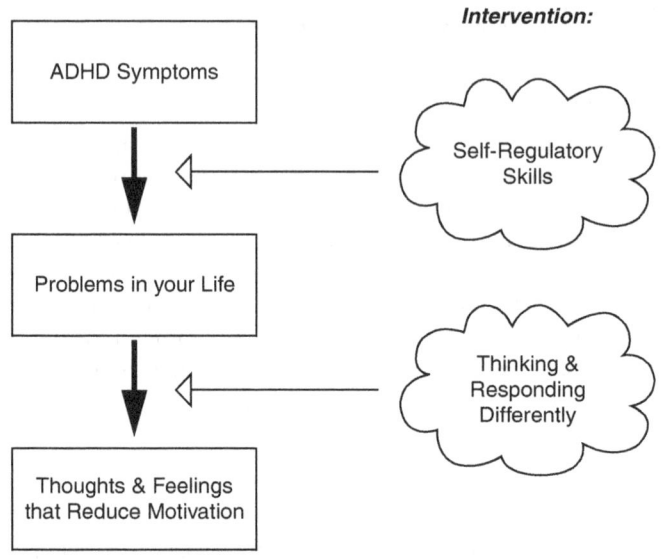

Figure 1 Simplified model of CBT for adult ADHD.

Dialogue 1

Therapist: *So far, we've really been emphasizing how you can learn new skills to cope better with ADHD. Today we're going to address the way ADHD can affect your thoughts and beliefs about yourself and how that can play a role in what you feel and what you do. How do you think your experience of ADHD affects the way you think about yourself?*

Client: *Wow, that's a great question. I guess one thing is that I kind of expect that I'm going to not finish things or let other people down and then when it starts to happen, I'm like, "OMG, not again …" And then I get really down on myself about it.*

Therapist: *Sure – that makes sense to me. You've had these experiences where ADHD gets in the way and so your brain is like, "Well, that's probably going to be the way it is no matter what." That's what brains do – they try to predict the future based on the past. But then it can make you feel …..?*

Client: *Tired. Like it's not worth it to try again.*

Therapist: *Yes, I've heard that from clients with ADHD a lot. It's also been recognized by researchers who study the disorder. Let me draw a picture to explain.* (Sketches the cognitive model, as in Figure 1.) *So we know that ADHD isn't **caused** by the way you think. It's a neurobiological disorder that contributes to inattention and hyperactivity/ impulsivity that, in certain environments and situations, leads to problems. And the ADHD symptoms make it harder to actually use the self-regulation skills that could help with the ADHD symptoms.*

But now we're going to add something new to this model – the way a lifetime of ADHD can impact your thoughts about yourself. Let me use the example you gave – you have these experiences of ADHD impacting your capacity to get things done and keep your promises to others and this leads to thoughts like … (looks expectantly at client).

Client: *"I'm just going to let people down again. Why should I even bother? It's just the way I am."*

Therapist: (Writes these on the diagram.) *So, then when you're thinking those thoughts, what feelings come up? And what do you feel like doing?*

Client: *Giving up, I guess? I just don't want to deal with it again.*

Therapist: *So, is it fair to say you're not feeling super-motivated to try to make things better?*

Client: *That's fair.*

Therapist: *Okay, so I'm going to write "De-Motivating Thoughts" in this box. So this is kind of like the WORST motivational speaker or coach ever – "Why even bother?," or even, "It's not that big of a deal. You'll be fine." And then you're more likely to disengage from doing what you might need to do to make it better, which leads to …* (draws arrow back to "Problems" box).

Client: *Yeah … pretty depressing.*

Therapist: *I can see that. It kind of feels like a cycle that's hard to get out of.*

Client: *Yeah.*

Therapist: *So what we're going to try to do is figure out the situations where these thoughts and feelings are most likely to happen for you and then practice some new ways of rolling with them when they come up. It's not easy, but I've found that when clients can become more aware of these thoughts, they can learn new ways to get out of the loop, so to speak.*

Teach Functional Assessment Using the General CBT Model

Next, you will present a general cognitive model (see Figure 2) that the client can use to analyze the relations among their thoughts, feelings, and actions and guide them in analyzing some examples from their daily life (see Dialogue 2 & Figure 2).

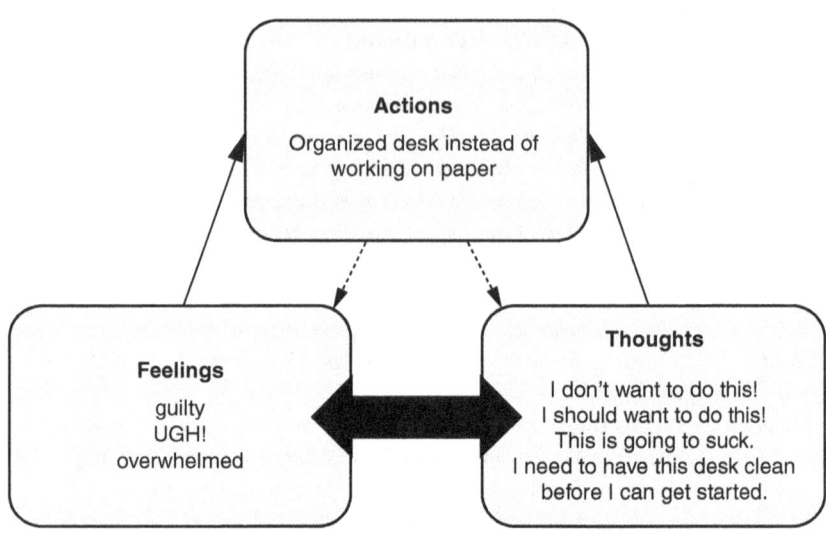

Figure 2 Thoughts-Feelings-Actions Model with Client Examples.

Dialogue 2

Therapist: Okay, we're going to use a simpler set-up to start to understand what happens for you when you're in a situation where you disengage from using skills. We're going to focus on how your thoughts, feelings, and actions might be related. (Draws general CBT diagram, like in Figure 2, as the example is reviewed.)

So, can you think of a time in the past week where you REALLY did not do what you intended to do with respect to getting things done or using a skill? Maybe, like, something you procrastinated on when you knew you shouldn't. (Therapist: Prompt client based on your knowledge of their biggest challenges).

Client: YES. I was supposed to be working on my paper ALL DAY yesterday and I just never did it. I just couldn't make myself.

Therapist: Okay, what were you doing instead?

Client: Anything else. Like, organizing my desk, for one thing.

Therapist: Okay. (Writes "organize desk instead of writing paper.") [***Note to therapist:*** You can start your teaching example with any of the three bubbles but it may be useful to work backward from a problematic avoidance response.]

So, right before you did that, what do you think you were thinking or feeling? If you can't remember exactly, give me your best guess based on what you know about yourself.

Client:	*Well, I felt bad that I wasn't doing what I was supposed to do.*
Therapist:	*Did that happen just before you worked on your desk?*
Client:	*Yeah, I think so.*
Therapist:	*Okay, cool.* (Writes "felt guilty" in "Feeling" bubble.) *Anything else you were feeling?*
Client:	*Yeah, just sort of an ... "UGH! I don't want to do this!" kind of a feeling.*
Therapist:	*I get that – it's hard to explain that feeling but I know what you're saying.* (Writes "UGH!" in the feeling bubble.) *And you mentioned maybe a thought in there – something you said to yourself. "I don't want to do this."* (Writes this in the thought bubble). *Anything else you were thinking just before you worked on the desk?*
Client:	*Yeah, I was thinking, "I SHOULD do this but I don't WANT to!"*
Therapist:	*Got it.* (Writes this in the thought bubble.) *Anything you might have thought about the task itself? Like about how it was going to go?*
Client:	*Yeah, I guess I probably thought that it was going to suck.*
Therapist:	*Let's write that down, too. And, based on what you said, I'm wondering if it's fair to say you might have been feeling ... overwhelmed?*
Client:	*Yeah, definitely add that.*
Therapist:	*Okay, cool. So I think you've painted a pretty detailed picture here for us to work with. So, in real life, it's hard to say which comes first – our thoughts or our feelings about things. Psychologists still haven't really figured that out but it's probably true that these things feed into one another.* (Draws back and forth arrows between feelings and thoughts bubble.) *Does that seem to fit your experience?*
Client:	*Yeah, it's hard to pull those apart, though.*
Therapist:	*Yes! And, when you're thinking all these things and feeling all these things, how motivated do you feel to work on the paper? Are you like, "HECK YEAH, let's get in there!?"*
Client:	*NO. More like get me out of here RIGHT NOW!*
Therapist:	*EXACTLY. You want to get away from those thoughts and feelings as quickly as possible and the easiest way to do that is to do ANYTHING ELSE other than work on the paper – to avoid, to distract yourself, to do something that's going to make you feel differently.* (Adds arrows from feelings and thoughts bubbles to action bubble.) *And so, in that moment, organizing your desk seems like a pretty logical response, at least in the short term. So, what did you think to yourself right before you started working on the desk?*
Client:	*Probably something like, "I need to have this desk clean before I can get started."*
Therapist:	*Gotcha. So you worked on the desk instead of the paper. How did that feel at first?*
Client:	*Sort of ... relief? I could distract myself from the paper and feel like I was accomplishing something.*
Therapist:	*So, it seemed like an okay choice in the moment. But what happened in the longer term?*

Client:	*Procrastination. The paper didn't get written, the problem didn't get dealt with. And I felt worse.*
Therapist:	(Adds arrows from Action to other bubbles.) *Right. And so what we need to do is help you develop some effective off-ramps for this cycle. Like I said, it's not easy, it's going to take some practice, but it is possible to get better at this over time. What do you think?*
Client:	*Seems like it could be overwhelming but ... seeing it all laid out here makes me feel like it might be possible.*

Present the Daily Thought Record (Self-monitoring Version)

Next, you will present and explain the self-monitoring version of the Daily Thought Record (DTR; see Table 1 and Appendix B). As with presenting the cognitive models, using examples from the client's life can help them to understand how to use this tool (see Dialogue 3).

Table 1 Daily Thought Record 1 – Self Monitoring Version

Situation – when and where?	Feelings	Thoughts	Action	Why was this action problematic?
In my dorm room; 10 pm on Sunday. Paper due tomorrow at 5 p.m.	guilty UGH! overwhelmed	I don't want to do this! I should want to do this! This is going to suck. I need to have this desk clean before I can get started.	Spent 45 min. organizing my desk	I needed to be working on my paper. Organizing the desk ended up making me feel worse in the long run.

Dialogue 3

Therapist:	*Next we'll need to get you more aware of how thoughts and feelings relate to actions in "real time." So, during this week, I'm going to have you do some self-monitoring, which is basically a fancy way of saying that you're going to track what's happening out in the real world. The purpose is to help you see patterns in how your thoughts, feelings, and actions relate to one another so you'll know what needs to change. Does that make sense?*
Client:	*I think so.*
Therapist:	(Presents the self-monitoring version of the DTR.) *So this chart takes the bubbles we just drew and turns them into columns. You're going to record*

> *some details about a situation in the first column, followed by what feelings you had, what thoughts you had, and what action you took - or maybe didn't take! Then, say a little something about why, looking back on it, that action led to problems.*

At this point, you ideally want to work through another example provided by the client in a similar manner to the dialogue in the previous section. You could use the same example as in the figure shown later or solicit a different example from the client, using the worksheet (see Appendix A). Try not to get too hung up on the order in which thoughts and feelings occurred, since these experiences are likely interactive. Instead, emphasize how they set the occasion for the problematic action.

Choose Targets for Self-monitoring and Define Homework

You will conclude the session by working with the client to set goals for using the DTR (see Appendix A) in self-monitoring as homework. In order to set the client up for success, you will decide on a specific homework target and discuss possible barriers and troubleshooting strategies.

Barriers to Self-monitoring

Begin assigning homework by asking the client what will get in the way of completing the DTR during the week. And, given the potential de-motivating influence of avoidant patterns of thinking, they may be particularly important to identify and address in a treatment like cognitive-behavioral therapy, which relies on the idea that adults with ADHD can, in fact, learn skills to improve self-regulation. Fortunately, there is some preliminary evidence that a growth mindset about self-regulation may be related to more adaptive emotional and behavioral responses to self-regulation challenges – even for people with higher levels of ADHD symptoms (Oddo et al., 2020). As such, therapists should consistently **support a growth mindset about self-regulation skills** – that is, they should convey the idea that, although genuinely difficult, acquisition of skills is possible with repeated practice and a willingness to try different strategies.

When to Complete the Form

Some cognitive approaches recommend that clients complete the form when they notice there has been a significant emotional shift. For clients with ADHD, however, another particularly important trigger might be when the client realizes that they have taken – or not taken – some kind of action that caused problems: such as getting distracted by another activity, putting off a necessary action, or not using a self-regulation tool (e.g., planner, task list). Help the client to generate some example instances that might be appropriate for self-monitoring.

When the client recognizes an appropriate instance, they should fill out the DTR as soon as they can in order to capture the experience. Alternatively, the client could set reminders in their phone or calendar app at strategic times per day and then, at the alarm, complete a DTR for instances that they can recall earlier in the day. If clients are concerned that they may not recall in detail the thoughts or feelings they had, they can be encouraged to make their best guess and mark on the form when their entries are assumptions rather than recollections.

DTR Format

Discuss with the client what format will be the most convenient for them – one that they will have easy access to. Some clients may prefer the paper handout while others may prefer to keep a copy in their task list or planner and then jot down the contents of each column on a blank notes page. Other clients may prefer to copy the form into a notes app on their phone.

Homework Goal

With the client, set a specific but realistic goal of the number of instances of self-monitoring to gather with the DTR over the course of the week. If the client sets an overly optimistic goal (e.g., completing the DTR every day five times per day), gently suggest a more reasonable goal. Emphasize that the goal of self-monitoring is to help the client practice becoming aware of the relation between thoughts, feelings, and actions in "real time" and to provide material to discuss in the next session.

Discuss Homework and Schedule Next Session

As described earlier, the homework for the week is for the client to use the DTR (see Appendix A) to record and analyze multiple examples of thoughts and feelings associated with problematic actions (or inactions). Ideally, they will record these details for use in the following week's session. As illustrated in the previous dialogue, be sure to set a specific and realistic target and discuss specifics of how the client will implement self-monitoring over the coming week.

References

Beck, J.S. (2011). *Cognitive behavior therapy: Basics and beyond* (Second Edition). Guilford Press.
Burnette, J.L., Babij, A.D., Oddo, L.E., & Knouse, L.E. (2020). Self-regulation mindsets: Relationship to coping, executive functioning, and ADHD. *Journal of Social and Clinical Psychology, 39*, 101–116. 10.1521/jscp.2020.39.02.101

Session 3: Practicing New Responses

Corresponds to Module 3.3 in the *Thriving in College* Student Workbook

Session Outline

1 Check-in with client(s)
2 Set agenda
3 Review homework – client examples from the DTR
4 Functional assessment
5 Identify red flag thoughts
6 Discuss effective coaching
7 Present the daily thought record (new responses version)
8 Practice generating alternative responses
9 Choose target situations for practice
10 Set homework
11 Schedule next session

Session Organization

Administration Format

The purpose of Session 3 is to help the client begin to practice new cognitive and behavioral responses in instances in which they have discovered that they are vulnerable to avoidant or otherwise problematic responses. As with Session 2, many clients will need more than one session to solidify these skills and all clients will need support to continue to practice engaging in new cognitive and behavioral responses throughout the remainder of the treatment. For the content in this session, in particular, clients may need more than one week of practice, and so this session may be repeated if that course of action suits your client's clinical needs.

Materials Needed

Use a whiteboard, flipchart, or a projected/shared digital document to work through client examples. You should also provide clients access to paper or

DOI: 10.4324/9781003149590-16

electronic handouts of Version 2 (new responses version) of the Daily Thought Record (see Appendix A).

Session Content
Check-in with Client(s)

Use this time to solicit brief discussion, or simply to see how things are going and build rapport. In the event that this session is the first meeting with clients, check-in might focus more on feelings and expectations about therapy. In any event, aim for this to be brief (< 5 minutes), encouraging for any additional discussion of this sort to be postponed until after the session content is completed. See therapist-client check-in dialogue example in Skill 1: Session 1 as a model for this interaction, if needed. We also recommend having your client complete the *Progress Tracker* (see Appendix B), and briefly touching base on any declines or improvements in school functioning.

Set Agenda

Introduce the agenda for this session to the client (see Session Outline). It may be helpful to have a visual aid to refer to, such as a flip chart or projected PowerPoint slide or printed handout. At this time it might also be helpful to remind clients to write notes regarding important points in a therapy notebook. Setting the agenda should be speedily completed (< 2 minutes). See therapist-client agenda-setting dialogue example in Skill 1: Session 1 as a model, if needed.

Review Homework from Previous Session

Referring to your notes and the prior module completed, briefly remind the client what their homework assignment was and discuss successes and barriers to completion. Carefully listen to their account of the situations that arose and how things went, as you will need to use the self-monitoring information the client(s) collected to engage them in functional analysis (see later).

Functional Assessment

You will collaboratively engage the client in a *functional assessment* – or an analysis of the factors that drive problematic responses. In traditional behavior analysis, functional assessment involves defining the target behavior and identifying the contingencies that might be maintaining it. Our approach to functional assessment includes an evaluation of the possible role of feelings and thoughts in prompting problematic behaviors, and an assessment of potential reinforcing consequences of subsequent thoughts and actions, as well.

As such, we take a functional approach to thoughts in that we consider them private behaviors that increase in frequency if they result in reinforcing consequences. As is the case for anxiety disorders and depressive disorders, the reinforcing consequences of problematic thoughts and behaviors can be described as **escape from aversive situations,** which include distressing or uncomfortable emotions and aversive tasks. In this sense, such thoughts and actions are maintained by **negative reinforcement**. For example, when a student with ADHD is trying to work on a term paper, but then gets a text from a friend about a party, a thought like "oh, I can finish this tomorrow, I can go out now" and the related behavior of interrupting their work is more likely to occur again in the future because these allow the student to *escape* the difficult task.

In sum, the goal of the functional assessment is to identify possible functional relations between feelings, thoughts, and actions that can serve as the basis for "doing things differently," or deviating from clients' use of adaptive behaviors and strategies. In addition, we want our clients to develop the skill of conducting their own functional assessments so that they can flexibly respond to the challenges that arise in daily life.

You should use examples from the client's self-monitoring homework to engage them in a discussion about the relations between their thoughts, feelings, and actions – particularly when they are experiencing self-regulation problems or procrastination. It can be helpful to refer to the latter as "avoidance mode," or to solicit from the client their own terminology for instances where thoughts and actions are causing significant disruption in meeting their goals.

If the client comes to the session without any self-monitoring data, first assess barriers to homework completion and make a plan for how the client could use previously learned skills for future homework, such as scheduling the task in their calendar, using When-Then contingencies, or setting reminders. Next, use the Daily Thought Record (Self-Monitoring Version) to elicit a few examples that can be used for the functional assessment. (If the aforementioned barriers to homework completion make good examples, use them!) See the prior module for sample dialogue and instructions on how to teach this skill.

Identifying Possible "Red Flag" Thoughts

Sometimes, clients have recurring thoughts that are associated with their problematic escape and avoidance responses. Explain to the client that, if they can become aware of the thoughts that often accompany "avoidance mode," then they have a better chance of responding differently (see Dialogue 1; Knouse & Mitchell, 2015). Importantly, these Red Flag Thoughts may not be overtly negative in content. Although some demotivating thoughts are certainly negative and pessimistic (e.g., "It's just not worth it to try anymore"), others may seem relatively neutral ("I can do that later"), or even positive and optimistic ("I do my best work under pressure, so I shouldn't really do this now"). Emphasize to the client that the most important feature of Red Flag Thoughts is their *function*, meaning whether they seem to be associated with "avoidance mode" vs. use of proactive self-regulation skills.

Dialogue 1

Therapist: *Interesting. So, in the two examples we've gone over today, I notice that you happen to have had the thought, "I'm too tired to do this." Is that a common thought for you?*

Client: *Yeah, I think so. Especially in the evening.*

Therapist: *And what tends to happen when you have that thought?*

Client: *I don't do whatever it is I'm thinking about, usually.*

Therapist: *Okay, so your motivation is low and you just put off doing the task and this isn't just a one time thing, it sounds like a pattern we're noticing here. I'm going to suggest that maybe the thought, "I'm too tired to do this." is what we call a Red Flag Thought for you. It signals that you're likely to avoid dealing with whatever it is you need to do right then. You're about to enter "avoidance mode," in other words. Does that seem fair?*

Client: *Yeah, I think so. But I really am tired when I think that.*

Therapist: *Sure! I hear that. That may be true for you. For now we're just looking for signals that you might be in avoidance territory so you can choose how you might want to respond instead of being on "autopilot." So, the thought, "I'm too tired to do this" could be a signal that there's a different way to respond.*

Client: *Ahh, okay, got it.*

Note that, in traditional cognitive restructuring, at this point the therapist might have engaged the client in a more extensive evaluation of the accuracy of the thought, "I'm too tired to do this," especially when the client raised the issue of accuracy. Instead, at this stage we recommend that you keep the focus of the conversation on the possible *function* of the thought, or the type of response it is associated with (Knouse & Mitchell, 2015).

If you and your client are unable to identify any recurrent avoidance thoughts that may be candidates for Red Flag Thoughts, simply proceed with the next step using a specific example from the client's Daily Thought Record homework.

Alternative Coaching

Next, you will use a metaphor to explain different ways the client could respond to the thoughts, feelings, and situations associated with "avoidance mode." The coaching metaphor presented here is based on the technique used by Safren and colleagues (2017) and expands upon the metaphor by including the idea of an overly permissive, optimistic, or unhelpful response to avoidance-related situations (see Dialogue 2 for an example). The purpose of this discussion is to help the client understand the different ways they could respond or "coach themselves" in situations where they are pulled toward avoidance and to identify the qualities of responses that are likely to help them engage in more adaptive behaviors.

Engage the client in a Socratic discussion[1] of their experiences with effective coaches or teachers in their lives. Inquire about the qualities of someone who was effective in motivating the client(s) and helping them build skills. Through your dialogue, highlight the qualities of effective coaching outlined in Box 1.

Dialogue 2

Therapist: I think one helpful way to think about how what you think and feel impacts your actions is to think about the way you might be coaching yourself. A coach's job is to motivate and teach the person they're coaching to perform more effectively. I'm curious if you've ever had experiences with effective and ineffective coaches or teachers?

Client: Yeah, definitely! I had this band teacher in high school who would just explode if you made a mistake. He was a total jerk and most kids hated him.

Therapist: Did he help you become a better musician?

Client: I mean, I guess I practiced more because I didn't want to get yelled at but I also was so petrified during practice that I started to hate it. I ended up dropping out of band.

Therapist: Yikes! So, is it fair to say that being overly harsh wasn't very motivating for you? Like, to the point that you didn't even want to try anymore?

Client: Yes, definitely.

Therapist: Do you think you ever coach yourself that way?

Client: Huh, I never really thought about that but ... yeah, I guess sometimes. Sometimes I might be like, "Why do you even try? You'll just screw it up."

Therapist: And I wonder if that possible Red Flag Thought is part of that? Like, "I'm WAY too tired to even try this." And when you think that you feel ....?

Client: Like why even bother trying.

Therapist: So it seems like a good coach at least has to be encouraging sometimes. They can't be 100% negative or it's just going to make you want to give up. Okay, so what if your band director had just been like, "You know what? All of you guys are amazing. Don't stress out about band too much and, if you need to, just take time for yourself instead of practicing. We can always rehearse next week."

Client:	*Ha! I had a softball coach like that. He wanted to be the "cool guy" all the time and let us get away with all kinds of slacking off.*
Therapist:	*Were you guys any good?*
Client:	*No! It was fun for a while but then we were, like, the worst team in the league and that sucked.*
Therapist:	*So, it also seems fair to say that a good coach has to call out what's not working and have some standards, even if they're going to be encouraging?*
Client:	*Yeah, I think they have to be able to have some structure and tell you what's not working or when you need to shape up.*
Therapist:	*Do you ever coach yourself like that lax softball coach? Like, I wonder if the example you came up with in your Daily Thought Record sort of fits here, too. "I'm too tired so … I can just rest for a few minutes. I deserve to take a break."*
Client:	(Laughs.) *Yes, definitely! When I don't want to do something it's easy for me to let things slide.*
Therapist:	*Okay, so a good coach has to be encouraging but also kind of realistic about the situation and what's not working well. So what if they just said, "Hey, your batting technique is off. Do better. Try harder. Just do it."*
Client:	*What if I don't know what exactly I'm doing wrong or how to do it right?*
Therapist:	*Exactly. So, in a way, a good coach has to be a good teacher, too. They need to tell you which strategies to use to improve, what to actually DO differently. Okay, so thanks for going through that little exercise with me. What do you think was the point of what we were talking about?*
Client:	*So, it seems like the way I've been coaching myself isn't always very helpful to doing what I want to do.*
Therapist:	*I think that's fair. Let's review the three things we're going to look for in good self-coaching.*

At this point, you should review the three aspects of good coaching outlined in the box given earlier. Next, you will apply these ideas to helping the client develop an alternative response.

Developing New Responses

In this step, you will help the client practice developing alternative cognitive and behavioral responses to example situations from the Daily Thought Record homework. If possible, continue to use key examples you have been focusing on throughout the session.

First, present and explain the Daily Thought Record – Alternative Response Version (see Appendix A). With the client, fill in the first four columns (Situation, Feelings, Thoughts, Actions) using an example from last week's homework. Next, engage the client in a discussion of why the action they took (or did not take) caused problems for them. Finally, collaborate with the client to formulate different ways they could coach themselves (i.e., think about the situation) and how they could respond differently. Guide the client in formulating responses that are **positive yet realistic** and responses that are **strategic** – especially those using skills the client has developed earlier in treatment (see Box 1).

In helping the client develop alternative cognitive and behavioral responses, the following questions may be useful:

- How could you have coached yourself more effectively?
- What is a more (encouraging, realistic) way of coaching yourself?
- What could you have done differently in this situation?
- Which other skills that we've worked on before could have been used here?
- How would you coach your best friend through this situation? (as in Table 1)

Box 1   A Good Coach

Encouraging: An effective coach doesn't berate you to the point of making you feel like there's no point in trying. Instead, they inspire you with the possibility that you can do better. They understand that progress takes time.

Realistic: On the other hand, an effective coach doesn't ignore the reality of what's <u>not</u> working. They don't ignore the problems you're having just to make you feel better. They understand that making you aware of what's going wrong is an important part of helping you improve.

Gives Good Strategies: An effective coach doesn't just identify what's not working and give you vague encouragement to "do better:" They suggest alternative techniques and help you practice those techniques until you can do them well.

Practicing New Responses

For homework this week, the client will practice formulating and, if possible, following through on new responses to challenging avoidance thoughts or situations. It may be helpful to identify specific problematic situations or Red Flag Thoughts that the client will focus on in the coming week, although they should be encouraged to use the Daily Thought Record to help formulate and practice new responses to any problematic situations they encounter (see Dialogue 3 for an example). The following dialogue illustrates how to direct a client's focus to a Red Flag Thought and how to encourage an empirical and exploratory approach to practicing new responses.

Table 1 Daily Thought Record 2 Example – Alternative Response Version

Situation – when and where?	Feelings	Thoughts	Action	Why was this action problematic?	Alternative coaching and actions
9:00 at night in my apartment. Saw the dishes piled up in the sink. Had promised my partner I'd take care of them this week.	Exhausted, overwhelmed. A little annoyed.	I am too tired to do this. I've been working ALL DAY. I'm just going to watch TV for a few minutes and then get started.	Watched Nexflix until I fell asleep on the couch.	I watched for longer than I wanted to and didn't get to the dishes. I woke up on the couch feeling terrible, like I let my partner down. Again.	Getting started is ALWAYS the worst part but it'll feel great to have them DONE. I could have propped my phone up on the window sill and watched Netflix while I did the dishes. Or put on a podcast.

Dialogue 3

Therapist: *Your goal this week is going to be to use this new set of steps to formulate new ways of coaching yourself and responding. It would be wonderful if you could actually carry out your new responses but, if you miss an opportunity, it's still helpful to think about alternative ways you could have responded. And, just to focus things a little more, I wonder if maybe we could really focus on time when you have that Red Flag Thought from earlier: "I'm just too tired to do this."*

Client: *So, you mean think of an alternative response when I have that thought?*

Therapist: *Yes! You can absolutely use the chart at other times, but for this week, I wonder what you'd think about focusing on that thought in particular?*

Client: *Okay, but what if I really am tired?*

Therapist: *Oh, I definitely think there are times when you'll feel tired and not end up changing your response, and that's okay. The goal here is to practice a different way to coach yourself and think of different ways you could respond. To give yourself the option of doing something different, at least. There may be times where you feel too tired, but it ends up you can still meet your goal anyway. Do you think that's true sometimes?*

Client: *Yeah, sometimes if I get going it's not too bad. I see what you're saying now.*

Discuss Homework and Schedule Next Session

As described earlier, the homework for the week is for the client to use the DTR – Alternative Responses Version (see Appendix A) to practice developing and following through on new coaching and responses to challenging avoidance situations. Many clients may benefit from multiple sessions that systematically focus on specific challenging situations and patterns of thinking. As such, you may decide to repeat the process of Session 3 for as many weeks as needed. In addition, if the client has completed other sessions in this module, you may want to assign repeated practice of the associated skills (e.g., mindfulness) as well.

Note

1 Socratic discussion is when a teacher asks open-ended questions and the learner, in answering, is able to contemplate their response and learn from it, something that is actively facilitated by the teacher. Of course, this is a process that you already know is central to psychotherapy.

References

Knouse, L.E., & Mitchell, J.T. (2015). Incautiously Optimistic: Positively Valenced Cognitive Avoidance in Adult ADHD. *Cognitive and Behavioral Practice*, *22*(2), 192–202. 10.1016/j.cbpra.2014.06.003

Safren, S.A., Sprich, S.E., Perlman, C.A., & Otto, M.W. (2017). *Mastering your adult ADHD: A Cognitive-Behavioral Treatment Program, Therapist Guide (treatments that work) 2nd Edition*. Oxford.

Session 4: Managing Strong Emotions and Impulsive Behavior

Corresponds to Module 3.4 in the *Thriving in College* Student Workbook

Session Outline

1 Check-in with client(s)
2 Set agenda
3 Review homework
4 Psychoeducation: impulsivity and strong emotions
5 Assessment of situational and emotional triggers for impulsivity
6 Choose targets and develop new responses
7 Visualization and covert rehearsal of new responses
8 Discuss emotion maintenance strategies
9 Set homework
10 Schedule next session

Session Organization

Administration Format

The purpose of Session 4 is to help the client develop and practice new cognitive and behavioral responses in situations that trigger strong emotions and impulsive behavior. Such scenarios call for advanced application of the cognitive and behavioral skills developed earlier in this module. We recommend that you spend ample time on the skills presented in Sessions 1 through 3 before proceeding with this module. As with prior sessions, this session may be repeated if that course of action suits your client's clinical needs.

Materials Needed

Use a whiteboard, flipchart, or a projected/shared digital document to work through client examples. Copies of the Daily Thought Record – Alternative Response Version (see Appendix A) will also be needed.

DOI: 10.4324/9781003149590-17

Session Content

Check-in with Client(s)

Use this time to solicit brief discussion, or simply to see how things are going and build rapport. In the event that this session is the first meeting with clients, check-in might focus more on feelings and expectations about therapy. In any event, aim for this to be brief (< 5 minutes), encouraging for any additional discussion of this sort to be postponed until after the session content is completed. See therapist-client check-in dialogue example in Skill 1: Session 1 as a model for this interaction, if needed. We also recommend having your client complete the *Progress Tracker* (see Appendix B), and briefly touching base on any declines or improvements in school functioning.

Set Agenda

Introduce the agenda for this session to the client (see Session Outline). It may be helpful to have a visual aid to refer to, such as a flip chart or projected PowerPoint slide or printed handout. At this time it might also be helpful to remind clients to write notes regarding important points in a therapy notebook. Setting the agenda should be speedily completed (< 2 minutes). See therapist-client agenda-setting dialogue example in Skill 1: Session 1 as a model, if needed.

Review Homework from Previous Session

Referring to your notes and the prior module completed, briefly remind the client what their homework assignment was and discuss successes and barriers to completion. In particular, carefully listen to their account of the situations that arose and note any situations in which strong emotions and impulsive behavior were problematic, as these examples can be used in discussions of the topics in this session.

Discuss Impulsivity and Strong Emotions in ADHD

Begin by engaging the client in a discussion of their experiences with difficulties regulating emotions and the impulsive behavior that is sometimes associated with it (see Dialogue 1 for an example). Briefly inform the client about the relation between ADHD and emotion dysregulation and its relation with impulsivity. In this discussion, we will discuss the idea of impulsivity in the presence of strong negative emotions such as anger, frustration, and anxiety (*negative urgency*) and in the presence of strong positive emotions such as excitement (*positive urgency*).

Dialogue 1

Therapist: *Today we're going to start to shift our focus a little bit and talk about times when you tend to act without thinking. Now that you've practiced coaching yourself differently and responding differently in several different situations, we're going to try to tackle what are probably the most challenging situations of all: those times when emotions can get you carried away and when it seems as though you act without thinking. Have there been any times like that for you in the past week?*

Client: *Yeah, definitely. Over the weekend, I got really mad at my friend and we had a huge fight. I said some really terrible stuff to them that I regretted later.*

Therapist: *Ugh, that's hard. It sounds like you felt really guilty afterwards for losing control. So, what happened? How did you get so mad?*

Client: *Well, we were at a party and playing a drinking game. They started to tease me and, at first, it was just fun but then they said something that REALLY made me mad and it reminded me of other times they said kinda crappy things to me. So I just went off and started yelling at them.*

Therapist: *Got it. So my guess is there were a couple of things going on. First, you had been drinking so we know that's always going to make you a little more impulsive, at least. But it sounds like it didn't just come out of nowhere – you felt something and thought something first, even though it probably seemed in the moment like your reaction came out of nowhere. You said you got mad remembering other crappy stuff they said to you?*

Client: *Yeah. I just got so pissed off all of a sudden.*

Therapist: *Gotcha. Makes sense because we know that in the presence of negative emotions like anger or frustration, people are prone to act more impulsively – that is, act without thinking. And, not only does alcohol make this emotional trigger more sensitive, but people with ADHD are often more prone to act without thinking when they're upset. Does that seem to fit your experience?*

Client: *Yeah, I've always had issues with my temper. And when I get super stressed out, my brain sort of shuts down, too.*

Therapist: *Sure. So we're going to try to work together to apply the coaching and new responses we've been working on to these times as well. But there's another thing I'm wondering about. What were you feeling earlier in the night when you started drinking?*

Client: *Oh, I felt great! I had just finished this huge project and turned it in so I was happy to be done with that and, on top of that, my team won in a huge come-from-behind game. So I was super excited to go out and celebrate all that.*

Therapist: *Got it. So, do you think feeling that good led to drinking more than you would have normally?*

> Client: *Maybe .... I've never thought about that.*
>
> Therapist: *So acting without thinking doesn't just increase when we are feeling really bad, but it can also happen when we're feeling really good. Has that been true for you in other situations?*
>
> Client: *Yeah, like when I'm with my friends and we're hyped about something, I did some really stupid stuff in high school — like risky stuff.*
>
> Therapist: *Got it. So as we work on this, we're going to pay attention to times when super positive emotions might contribute to you doing impulsive things that could cause trouble for you and also times that really negative emotions might do the same thing.*

Assess Emotional States and Situations Most Associated with Impulsivity

Next, work with the client to identify initial target emotional states and situations for developing new, non-impulsive responses. One strategy is to first assess whether the client experiences impulsivity in the presence of a particular category of affect, such as anxiety, frustration, anger, anticipation, or excitement. You can then choose to focus on the situations that are associated with that challenging emotion in the coming week. Next, solicit from the client what situations are most likely to elicit the challenging emotion and what their problematic impulsive responses tend to be.

An alternative strategy would be to identify the most problematic impulsive response – such as drinking alcohol, spending money, or lashing out at others – and use functional assessment to identify the situations and emotions in which the client is most vulnerable. In either case, your goal is to identify some specific situations and emotions that can be the target for skills practice in the coming week.

The Daily Thought Record can be very helpful in organizing information about these emotions and situations into a format that the client has become accustomed to. In any event, make sure to keep a written record of the client's input for reference later.

Choose Targets and Develop New Responses

When helping clients change impulsive responding, which can be quite challenging, start by focusing on some specific target situations and emotions that were identified in the previous step. Leaning on skills from Session 3: Practicing New Responses (see earlier) that the client has likely started to develop, work through some specific examples using the Daily Thought Record – Version 2 (Appendix A). In particular, help the client identify typical **Red Flag Thoughts** (see p. 125) associated with their challenging emotions and guide

Table 1 Daily Thought Record – Examples for Addressing Emotional Impulsivity

Situation – when and where?	Feelings	Thoughts	Action	Why was this action problematic?	Alternative coaching and actions
10:00 p.m. Monday – my friend sent me a snarky text	Mad, hurt, frustrated, a little sad 😠	She's lecturing me like I'm her kid, she's acting like she's better than me.	Sent snarky texts back Ghosted her for the rest of the night	I realized I overreacted. She didn't mean it like I thought I said a bunch of mean things I'm not proud of.	This is pissing me off but I know sometimes texts come across wrong, I'm going to put the phone down, do a 2-minute mindfulness exercise and then either do something else or just call her to work it out.
7:30 pm. Thursday	Hyped, excited. Relieved to be almost done with the week.	I can't really remember but probably just: Yeah! I deserve to have fun and not care about anything.	Spent an hour pre-partying in my friend's room and took a bunch of shots while playing a drinking game. Got way more drunk than I intended.	When we went out I got really disoriented and blacked out and my friends had to take me home and ruin their fun, which sucked. I woke up SOOO hung over and missed rehearsal.	To have the maximum possible fun I need to NOT overdo it like last time! I'm going to skip drinking games tonight, tell my friends that in advance, and keep it to two beers before we go out.

them in developing **alternative coaching** (see p. 126) that is **encouraging, realistic**, and that suggests **good strategies**. See Table 1 for some examples of new responses a client might develop for situations that make them vulnerable to anger-impulsivity as well as impulsivity that seems cued by strong positive emotion.

Visualization Practice of New Responses

Explain that, by definition, impulsive responding happens in a way that feels automatic and *without* forethought. Therefore, it is helpful to have *even more practice* responding to situations and emotions that can trigger impulsivity than might be the case for other kinds of new responses. To provide the opportunity for more practice, you will work together to practice responses by visualizing the situation and the thoughts and feelings that make it difficult to resist impulsive responding in "real life," which you identified in the previous step.

Begin to engage your client in visualization practice by referring to your previous work with the client on mindfulness (see Dialogue 2). You may wish to use a short deep breathing or body scan script to help the client settle their mind and engage with the exercise. Next, lead the client through visualization of the key situation that they will be targeting for practice this week. Engage them in sensing what surrounds them in the trigger situation and how their body feels. Elicit the impulsivity-related trigger thoughts that occur in the moment and guide them in responding to those thoughts and emotions with alternative coaching and visualization of the alternative coping response. Depending on the time available, you may repeat this exercise during the session, perhaps slightly altering the situation or trigger to match other possible settings in which the client may be vulnerable to.

Dialogue 2

Therapist: Okay, now I'm going to ask you to go back in your mind to the incident from this past week when you argued with your friend over text. Take a moment to place yourself in the physical space where you were when you got the text. Where are you? What does it look like?

Client: I'm in my dorm room sitting at my desk. The room is dark with just my desk lamp on and the light from my laptop screen.

Therapist: Great. Take a moment and really feel like you're back there in your room. What does it feel like and what sounds do you hear?

Client: It's a little chilly so I have my hoodie on. The heat keeps cutting on and making a noise every time.

Therapist: Great. What are you doing?

Client:	*I'm trying to write a response paper for my poli sci class. I just can't get started, though. I'm just kind of staring at the screen zoning out.*
Therapist:	*Okay, stay with that feeling. Then the text arrives. How do you know you've gotten it?*
Client:	*My phone buzzes. I pick it up and see it's a text from Maddie.*
Therapist:	*Read it out loud.*
Client:	*She says, "Hey, do you want to come over now?"*
Therapist:	*What do you feel? What do you say to yourself?*
Client:	*Just, "UGH!" I can't come over and she knows it because I told her I have work to do.*
Therapist:	*What do you do?*
Client:	*I text back: "Can't. Haven't finished my work yet." And she texts back, "GIRL. I thought you started at, like, 5. Why r u not done yet?"*
Therapist:	*What do you feel in your body when you read that?*
Client:	*Just … my chest gets tight, I tense up. I feel SO PISSED. She KNOWS I am having a hard time and she's flippin' LECTURING me. AGAIN.*
Therapist:	*Okay, and so you … .*
Client:	*So I text back, "I guess SOME people actually care about their grades," and then a winky emoji.*
Therapist:	*And you felt …*
Client:	*Satisfied. Until she texted back.*

At this point, you might pause the scene and briefly review the events that followed and their consequences (see Dialogue 3). Alternatively, you might continue the visualization to other key moments of impulsive responding. When you have reviewed the most important moments when alternative responses could have led to a more adaptive outcome, begin the scene again and help the client covertly rehearse alternative responses.

Dialogue 3

[After rewinding the scene, the therapist works through the initial events, arriving at the point where the client receives the text.]

Client:	*She texts back, "GIRL. I thought you started at, like, 5. Why r u not done yet?"*
Therapist:	*What do you feel in your body?*
Client:	*I tense up. I feel pissed.*
Therapist:	*Are you feeling it now?*
Client:	*Yes.*
Therapist:	*Good. And your mind says … .?*

Client:	She *KNOWS* how hard it is for me and she thinks it's her right to lecture because she thinks she's *BETTER* than me.
Therapist:	Good, it's okay to feel that anger but it doesn't have to dictate what you do. You don't have to like what's happening, but you have a choice. How do you coach yourself in that moment?
Client:	Okay... uhhh ... maybe: Ugh! She can be SO annoying sometimes. I *REALLY* want to text back but I can feel how mad I am and I'm just going to say something dumb. Lemme just put the phone away and breathe or walk around for a minute.
Therapist:	Good – envision yourself feeling angry and laying the phone down, maybe sticking it in a drawer. Taking a deep breath. Go ahead and do that now – deep breaths. Get a sense of feeling the anger but breathing through it. And then tell me about your thoughts.
Client:	(Takes a few deep breaths.) *I'm still annoyed. I just can't respond right now. I'll text her later.*
Therapist:	Good – that sounds like it was a hard moment.

At this point, the therapist and client can repeat the covert rehearsal, possibly imagining and practicing other ways of coaching and coping. After completing the visualizations, you should debrief the experience with the client and identify any additional coaching or coping "nuggets" that emerged from the experience that could be useful in real-world practice.

Emotion Maintenance Strategies

In addition to targeted practice for vulnerable moments, some clients may benefit from the regular use of strategies and lifestyle choices that promote emotion regulation. For example, healthy eating, regular exercise, and adequate sleep, which are emphasized elsewhere in this program, can prevent the emotional dysregulation that can result from a depleted body. Emotion Regulation and Distress Tolerance skills included in Dialectical Behavior Therapy Skills Training (Linehan, 2014) may provide additional ideas for practices that promote emotion regulation. Discuss with the client what factors promote emotion regulation and dysregulation for them and consider assigning these healthy practices for homework.

Set Homework

Work with the client to identify times when they might be likely to encounter their trigger situations or emotions during the week and collaboratively plan to use their Daily Thought Record to process and respond to these situations. Emphasize that these are likely to be the most challenging situations in which to practice new responses, so it's a good idea to be very specific about the situations that are problematic and to plan. Normalize the experience of responding impulsively despite their intention and instruct them to complete their record as soon as they can after the event and bring it to the next session to discuss. Next, assign the client to practice visualizing and responding to their trigger situation at a regular frequency over the course of the next week and, as always, assess barriers to homework completing and plan for implementation. Finally, assign specific homework related to any emotion maintenance strategies discussed during the session, if applicable.

Reference

Linehan, M.M. (2014). *DBT Skills Training Manual, Second Edition.* Guilford.

Skill 4: Taking Good Care of Yourself

(~3 sessions)

Corresponds to Skillset 4 of the *Thriving in College* Student Workbook

Background for the Therapist

A strong link has been found between mental health and physical health. For example, negative affect has been shown to be predictive of coronary heart disease in adult men and women (Nabi et al., 2008) and emotional distress is associated with risk of stroke (Surtees et al., 2008) in this same population. Researchers have proposed several pathways through which mental health problems can lead to physical health difficulties, including through poor decision making, unhealthy lifestyle choices, reduced social connections, or loss of employment (Ohrnberger et al., 2017). Although the mechanisms supporting the links between physical health and various mental health problems differ, we will focus here on the literature supporting the links between healthy lifestyle behaviors and ADHD. Specifically, we will consider how ADHD in college students can impact physical well-being and vice versa.

There are several areas of physical well-being that are frequently impacted by ADHD symptoms and can also contribute to symptom severity. Some or all of these areas may be of concern to college students participating in this intervention. In the sessions that follow, we first present background psychoeducation on how ADHD is related to sleep, nutrition, physical activity, substance use, technology use, and safe driving. It is important to begin with this background so that clients understand the context for discussing strategies to improve in these areas. Next, we provide guidance on how to help the student client identify whether they would like to make changes in any of the six areas. Clients are also encouraged to engage in goal-setting around the chosen areas. Finally, building from the OTMP skills taught earlier in this intervention, we introduce a series of strategies for improving sleep, eating healthier, increasing physical activity, managing substance and technology use, and driving safely. Students are encouraged to select several strategies to incorporate in their routines.

Although the psychoeducation can be presented in a group format, the remainder of the sessions in this module should be conducted with each client

DOI: 10.4324/9781003149590-18

individually because the identification of target areas and specific strategies a client selects will likely vary by client. Examples of dialogue between the therapist and client are provided for Sessions 2 and 3.

Student Workbook

If you are using the *Thriving in College* student workbook, you will find that Skillset 4 on *Taking Good Care of Yourself* corresponds to the material in this section. In this therapist guide, we recommend that you provide psychoeducation (Session 1) and then assess your client's specific needs for health and lifestyle skills (Session 2) and tailor the content you emphasize accordingly. As such, Session 3 in the manual corresponds to multiple modules in the workbook, allowing you to tailor skills information and skills practice opportunities to each client.

Therapist Guide Session	Workbook Modules
1	4.0 Why it Matters, Pre-Assessment, and Roadmap
2 and 3	4.1 Sleeping Better
	4.2 Eating Healthier
	4.3 Increasing Physical Activity
	4.4 Managing Substance Abuse
	4.5 Managing Technology Use
	4.6 Driving Safely

References

Nabi, H., Kivimaki, M., De Vogli, R., Marmot, M.G., & Singh-Manoux, A. (2008). Positive and negative affect and risk of coronary heart disease: Whitehall II prospective cohort study. *British Medical Journal, 337*(7660), 32–36. 10.1136/bmj.a118

Ohrnberger, J., Fichera, E., & Sutton, M. (2017). The relationship between physical and mental health: A mediation analysis. *Social Science & Medicine, 195*, 42–49. 10.1016/j.socscimed.2017.11.008

Surtees, P.G., Wainwright, N.W., Luben, R.N., Wareham, N.J., Bingham, S.A., & Khaw, K.T. (2008). Psychological distress, major depressive disorder, and risk of stroke. *Neurology, 70*(10), 788–794. 10.1212/01.wnl.0000304109.18563.81

Session 1: How is ADHD Related to Sleep, Nutrition, Physical Activity, Substance Use, Technology Use, and Driving?

Corresponds to Module 4.0 in the *Thriving in College* Student Workbook

Session Outline

1 Check-in with client(s)
2 Set agenda
3 Review homework
4 How is ADHD related to sleep?
5 How is ADHD related to nutrition?
6 How is ADHD related to physical activity?
7 How is ADHD related to substance use?
8 How is ADHD related to technology use?
9 How is ADHD related to driving?
10 Discuss homework
11 Schedule the next session

Session Organization

Administration Format

Session 1 can be administered in a group or individual format. A group session may work well for delivering psychoeducation about ADHD and healthy lifestyles and giving clients the opportunity to discuss their experiences.

Materials Needed

You should bring a whiteboard, flipchart, or projected document to capture group ideas (as warranted by the format used). Attending students should have a notebook or pad of paper to take notes.

Session Content

Check-in with Client(s)

Use this time to solicit brief discussion, or simply to see how things are going and build rapport. If this session is the first meeting with clients, check-in might

DOI: 10.4324/9781003149590-19

focus more on feelings and expectations about therapy. In any event, aim for this to be brief (< 5 minutes), encouraging for any additional discussion of this sort to be postponed until after the session content is completed. See therapist-client check-in dialogue example in Skill 1: Session 1 as a model for this interaction, if needed. We also recommend having your client complete the *Progress Tracker* (see Appendix B), and briefly touching base on any declines or improvements in school functioning.

Set Agenda

Introduce the agenda for this session to the client (see Session Outline). It may be helpful to have a visual aid to refer to, such as a flip chart or projected PowerPoint slide or printed handout. At this time, it might also be helpful to remind clients to write notes regarding important points in a therapy notebook. Setting the agenda should be speedily completed (< 2 minutes). See therapist-client agenda-setting dialogue example in Skill 1: Session 1 as a model, if needed.

Review Homework from Previous Session

Referring to your notes and the prior module completed, briefly remind the client what their homework assignment was and discuss successes and barriers to completion. Carefully listen to their account of the situations that arose and note any situations in which strong emotions and impulsive behavior were problematic.

In this session, we will discuss how ADHD symptoms can impact and be impacted by six areas of physical well-being, including sleep, nutrition, physical activity, substance use, technology use, and driving. It is important to begin with this background psychoeducation so that clients understand the context for discussing strategies to improve these areas in the sessions that follow. Because this initial session involves delivery of a great deal of information, you are encouraged to think about how to keep clients engaged during the session. For instance, it is recommended to begin each topic with a discussion of what the client already knows, and then transition into a presentation of new information you will find below. We strongly recommend reading this section thoroughly before meeting with your client, following up with additional reading on any interesting topics in more detail, as needed or desired.

How Is ADHD Related to Sleep?

It is estimated that between 25% and 50% of individuals with ADHD experience sleep problems, which includes shorter sleep time, difficulties falling and staying asleep, and a higher risk of developing a sleep disorder (Wajszilber et al., 2018). Scientists have hypothesized that these sleep problems may be due to differences in arousal, alertness, and regulation circuits in the brain, or to a delayed circadian rhythm cycle (Wajszilber et al., 2018). College students in general also often have poor sleep habits, including irregular bed- and wake-up-times, heavy substance use which can impact getting restorative sleep, variable sleep length from night to night, and regularly pulling "all-nighters" for studying or partying. These sleep habits can be exacerbated by having ADHD. Poor organization and time management skills mean that college students with ADHD may stay up late for last-minute studying or completing school as-signments. These students may also have difficulty transitioning to sleep from stimulating activities, such as playing video games. Additionally, as will be discussed later in this chapter, heavy substance use is more of a risk among college students with ADHD. Other disorders that often co-occur with ADHD, such as anxiety or depression, can also have a negative impact on sleep habits and patterns. Finally, stimulant medications that are often prescribed to treat ADHD (e.g., Adderall, Ritalin) may cause difficulty with falling asleep if taken too late in the day. Combined, these various risk factors result in many college students with ADHD getting inadequate sleep on a regular basis.

It is important to note that inadequate sleep can result in ADHD-like symptoms, such as difficulty concentrating, forgetfulness, and problems with maintaining focus, and can also make existing ADHD symptoms worse (Gloger & Suhr, 2020; Taylor et al., 2013). Daytime sleepiness and napping can result in college students with ADHD frequently missing classes or study time. This can lead to lower grades in classes and exacerbate existing academic impair-ments. Inadequate sleep can also cause irritability, which can impair the social relationships of college students with ADHD, which are sometimes already strained. Many college students with ADHD can benefit from taking measures to improve their sleep and sleep habits. In the next module, we will talk about several strategies for improving sleep.

How Is ADHD Related to Nutrition?

There has been a longstanding debate about whether diet might cause or contribute to ADHD. The scientific consensus is that diet does not cause ADHD and that sugar does not make children hyperactive (e.g., Hoover & Milich, 1994). Furthermore, dietary interventions (e.g., Feingold diet) have not been shown to be effective for the treatment of ADHD. Nonetheless, in the last five years, research has shown nutrition might impact the severity of ADHD symptoms over time and that some dietary interventions might be useful as adjunctive treatments. Stated differently, poor nutrition does not cause ADHD but it could exacerbate symptoms (see Nigg, 2017; *Getting Ahead of ADHD*).

According to Nigg (2018), there are a few important advances in recent years. First, omega-3 supplements (e.g., fish oil capsules) have been shown to reduce ADHD symptoms. This is now considered a reliable effect although not as large as that obtained from stimulant medication and/or behavior therapy. Therefore, fish oil supplements can be recommended as an adjunct to other well-established interventions. Second, decreasing one's intake of highly processed foods might improve ADHD symptoms in some people. Given that this recommendation is also good for general health, there is little risk in giving it a try. As mentioned previously, it has been shown that sugar intake does not immediately result in increased hyperactivity (e.g., when a child eats candy there are probably other aspects to the situation that are impacting activity levels such as the excitement of a birthday party or Halloween). However, more recent research suggests that poor nutrition over time may have a negative impact on attention and behavior. For this reason, Nigg (2018) recommends avoiding added sugar, saturated fats, caffeinated and energy drinks, and artificial food additives. There is also some research on the use of multi-nutrient supplements in ADHD (e.g., Rucklidge et al., 2017). Although multi-nutrient supplements might be a more accessible avenue to obtaining the benefits of a fresh food diet, this research is still too preliminary to recommend multi-nutrients widely.

A meta-analysis has shown a significant relation between ADHD and obesity (Cortese et al., 2015). Although a causal relation has not been established, Nigg (2018) has suggested several explanations including the possibility that those with ADHD may be engaging in more impulsive eating than their peers which puts them at greater risk for excess weight gain. Another factor that may contribute to poor eating habits in college students in general, and those with ADHD, is that healthy eating requires time management and planning skills (e.g., planning meals, going grocery shopping, and preparing food). Prior to college, students often rely on their parents to perform these tasks. Suddenly, when they begin college, and especially when they move out of the dorms and into an apartment, they are now entirely responsible for buying and preparing their own meals. For those with ADHD, who have more difficulty with organization, time management, and planning, there may be an even greater likelihood that meals are quickly prepared, grabbed from fast food restaurants, or skipped altogether, which might result in eating larger meals later or more junk food between meals.

How Is ADHD Related to Physical Activity?

There are several ways in which physical activity levels might be influenced by ADHD symptoms and vice versa. As with good sleep and nutrition, before describing these relations, it is worth mentioning that there are multiple benefits of physical activity more generally. Physical exercise has been shown to improve physical (e.g., cardiovascular disease, diabetes) and psychological (e.g., anxiety, depression) problems (see Hillman, Erickson & Kramer, 2008). Due to these benefits, the Centers for Disease Control (CDC, 2018) has recommended that adults engage in at least 150 minutes of moderate intensity exercise per week (e.g., 30 minutes × 5 days per week, 50 minutes × 3 days per week, 75 minutes × 2 days per week). However, only 23.2% of adults in the US meet these criteria (CDC, 2018). Thus, we are on solid ground for reiterating these CDC guidelines to all of our college student clients even though the evidence for the impact on ADHD is still preliminary.

In terms of the reciprocal relation between ADHD symptoms and physical exercise, there is preliminary evidence that physical exercise helps improve symptoms of ADHD. Specifically, acute positive effects on symptoms (i.e., immediately following a period of exercise) have been demonstrated in children and adolescents (see Neudecker et al., 2019 for a review) and emerging adults (Gapin et al., 2015). Furthermore, chronic effects (i.e., occurring after engaging in a regular exercise program) have been shown in a few studies with children who have ADHD (e.g., Hoza et al., 2015). There is also evidence that physical exercise helps with anxiety and depression (see Rebar et al., 2015 for a review), albeit through different mechanisms. Given that anxiety and depression are often comorbid in individuals with ADHD, physical exercise may have a plethora of benefits for college students with ADHD. Despite the potential positive benefits on physical and mental health, it may be especially challenging for college students with ADHD to establish a regular exercise routine. Specifically, poor organizational, time management, and planning skills may interfere with completing necessary tasks (e.g., schoolwork, housework) such that it may be even more difficult to make time for physical exercise. Furthermore, students with ADHD may have less motivation toward physical activity than students without ADHD (Serrano et al., 2022). Therefore, interventions may need to focus on multiple goals including increasing motivation toward physical exercise and improving time management skills to create time for exercise.

How Is ADHD Related to Substance Use?

Frequent and heavy substance use is common among college students. Compared to young adults who are not attending college, more college students report having been drunk during the past 30 days (35% vs. 28%) and binge drinking (i.e., drinking five or more drinks in a row) during the past two weeks (33% vs. 22%; Schulenberg et al., 2020). Twenty-six percent of college students report marijuana use during the past 30 days and students also use other illicit drugs, but to a lesser degree (Schulenberg et al., 2020).

Having ADHD can pose additional risks for substance use and problems associated with use for college students. ADHD in the college student population is strongly associated with heavy substance use and associated problems, particularly for alcohol, as well as related impairment (Rooney et al., 2012; Rooney et al., 2015). Other disorders that commonly co-occur with ADHD, such as anxiety and depression, can also pose an increased risk for substance use and problems associated with use (Lai et al., 2015). Finally, college students with symptoms of ADHD may misuse certain substances in order to manage their symptoms. This includes nicotine, caffeine, and prescription stimulant medication (e.g., Adderall, Ritalin). With regards to misuse of prescription stimulant medication, evidence suggests that both ADHD and depression symptoms are associated with this behavior (Benson & Flory, 2017).

Heavy and frequent substance use can have negative impacts on college students' physical and mental health, academic success, and social relationships. Misuse of alcohol or other substances can also result in symptoms that look like ADHD, such as difficulty concentrating and low motivation. In fact, evidence suggests that, in many cases, ADHD-like symptoms that first emerge during young adulthood can be better accounted for by heavy substance use (e.g., Sibley et al., 2017).

For all these reasons, many college students with ADHD may wish to more closely monitor and eventually reduce their use of alcohol, marijuana, or other substances. Some research evidence (Looby et al., 2019; Looby et al., 2021) also suggests that there are some very specific behavioral strategies that college students with elevated ADHD symptoms can engage in that may reduce problems associated with alcohol use, such as missing class, being hungover, DUIs, and other undesirable outcomes related to heavy use. These are called Protective Behavior Strategies. Examples of such strategies are setting a predetermined time to stop drinking and avoiding drinking games. In the next module, we will further discuss these behavioral strategies as well as other ways to reduce substance use and associated problems.

How Is ADHD Related to Technology Use?

Although some types of technology may be extremely helpful for individuals with ADHD (e.g., word processors, electronic calendars and task lists, phone reminders), research has shown that individuals with ADHD are at greater risk for excessive use of other types of technology (e.g., gaming, using social media, viewing video clips; Werling et al., 2021). More specifically, multiple studies have documented a strong relation between problematic gaming and ADHD in college students (e.g., Lefler et al., 2022) and other age groups (see Dullur et al. 2021 for a review).

In addition to the direct effects of technology on time management and procrastination, technology use may also impact the relation between ADHD and sleep. Individuals with ADHD have more sleep problems than those without ADHD. Research has shown that evening screen use impacts sleep quality in preschool children (Brockmann et al., 2016). Furthermore, a recent study by Cavalli et al. (2021) demonstrated that evening screen use in school-age children with ADHD is directly related to increased sleep problems (e.g., insomnia, breathing difficulties, non-restorative sleep). Thus, evening screen use is *even more* likely to cause sleep problems in those with ADHD. In addition,

Cavalli et al. (2021) found that evening screen exposure was also associated with increased attention problems during the day as a result of poorer sleep quality. Thus, there is good evidence that excessive technology use has a significant impact on productivity and sleep quality in college students with ADHD.

How Is ADHD Related to Driving?

Research also shows that college students and other adults with ADHD tend to have more impairment related to driving, as compared to peers without ADHD. Specifically, those with ADHD have more car accidents, get more speeding tickets, and have more overall driving-related citations (Barkley et al., 2002; Merkel et al., 2013). Those with ADHD also report less use of safe driving behaviors, more risky driving behaviors, more difficulties with concentration while driving, and more instances of anger while driving than individuals without the disorder (e.g., Richards et al., 2002). One study showed that people with ADHD had a profile of driving impairment similar to people without ADHD who were intoxicated at the legal limit in the U.S., suggesting that driving while under the influence of alcohol may be even more dangerous for people with ADHD (Weafer et al., 2008). Although taking stimulant medication consistently as prescribed can reduce these driving-related risks for those with ADHD (Barkley & Cox, 2007), there are also other behavioral strategies that can help.

Discuss Homework and Schedule Next Session

Prompt your client to think about whether any of these healthy lifestyle areas might be impacting, or impacted by, their ADHD symptoms. They should come prepared to discuss this in the next session.

References

Benson, K., & Flory, K. (2017). Symptoms of depression and ADHD in relation to stimulant medication misuse among college students. *Substance Use & Misuse, 52*(14), 1937–1945. 10.1080/10826084.2017.1318146

Brockmann, P.E., Diaz, B., Damiani, F., et al. (2016). Impact of television on the quality of sleep in preschool children. *Sleep Medicine, 20*, 140e4. 10.1016/j.sleep.2015.06.005

Barkley, R. A., Murphy, K. R., Dupaul, G. J., & Bush, T. (2002). Driving in young adults with attention deficit hyperactivity disorder: Knowledge, performance, adverse outcomes, and the role of executive functioning. *Journal of the International Neuropsychological Society, 8*, 655–67210.1017/s1355617702801345

Barkley, R. A., & Cox, D. (2007). A review of driving risks and impairments associated with attention-deficit/hyperactivity disorder and the effects of stimulant medication on driving performance. *Journal of Safety Research, 38*(1),113–128. 10.1016/j.jsr.2006.09.004

Cavalli, E., Anders, R., Chaussoy, L., Herbillon, V., Franco, P., & Putois. B. (2021). Screen exposure exacerbates ADHD symptoms indirectly through increased sleep disturbance. *Sleep Medicine, 83*, 241–247. 10.1016/j.sleep.2021.03.010

Centers for Disease Control and Prevention (2018). How much physical activity do adults need? *cdc.gov.* https://www.cdc.gov/physicalactivity/basics/adults/index.htm

Cortese, S., Ferrin, M., Brandeis, D., Buitelaar, J., Daley, D., Dittmann, R.W., Holtmann, M., Santosh, P., Stevenson, J., Stringaris, A., Zuddas, A., Sonuga-Barke, E.J., & European ADHD Guidelines Group (EAGG) (2015). Cognitive training for attention-deficit/hyperactivity disorder: meta-analysis of clinical and neuro-psychological outcomes from randomized controlled trials. *Journal of the American Academy of Child and Adolescent Psychiatry, 54*(3), 164–174. 10.1016/j.jaac.2014.12.010

Dullur, P., Krishnan, V., & Diaz, A.M. (2021). A systematic review on the intersection of attention-deficit hyperactivity disorder and gaming disorder. *Journal of Psychiatric Research, 133*, 212–222. 10.1016/j.jpsychires.2020.12.026

Gapin, J.I., Labban, J.D., Bohall, S.C., Wooten, J.S., & Chang, Y.K. (2015). Acute exercise is associated with specific executive functions in college students with ADHD: A preliminary study. *Journal of Sport and Health Science, 4*, 89–96. 10.1016/j.jshs.2014.11.003

Gloger, E.M., & Suhr, J.A. (2020). Correlates of poor sleep and subsequent risk of misdiagnosis in college students presenting with cognitive complaints. *Archives of Clinical Neuropsychology, 35*(6), 692–700. 10.1093/arclin/acaa023

Hillman, C., Erickson, K. & Kramer, A. (2008). Be smart, exercise your heart: exercise effects on brain and cognition. *Nature Reviews Neuroscience, 9*, 58–65. 10.1038/nrn2298

Hoover, D.W., & Milich, R. (1994). Effects of sugar ingestion expectancies on mother-child interactions. *Journal of Abnormal Child Psychology, 22*(4), 501–515. 10.1007/BF02168088

Hoza, B., Smith, A.L., Shoulberg, E.K., Linnea, K.S., Dorsch, T.E., Blazo, J.A., Alerding, C.M., & McCabe, G.P. (2015). A randomized trial examining the effects of aerobic physical activity on attention-deficit/hyperactivity disorder symptoms in young children. *Journal of Abnormal Child Psychology, 43*(4), 655–667. 10.1007/s10802-014-9929-y

Lai, H.M., Cleary, M., Sitharthan, T., & Hunt, G.E. (2015). Prevalence of comorbid substance use, anxiety and mood disorders in epidemiological surveys, 1990–2014: A systematic review and meta-analysis. *Drug and Alcohol Dependence, 154*, 1–13. 10.1016/j.drugalcdep.2015.05.031

Lefler, E.K., Alacha, H.F., Vasko, J.M., Serrano, J.W., Looby, A., Flory, K., & Hartung, C.M. (2022 in press). Sex differences in ADHD symptoms, problematic gaming, and impairment in college students. *Current Psychology.*

Looby, A., Bravo, A.J., Kilwein, T.M., Zimmerman, L., Pearson, M.R., & Protective Strategies Study Team (2019). Alcohol-related protective behavioral strategies as a mediator of the relationship between drinking motives and risky sexual behaviors. *Addictive Behaviors, 93*, 1–8. 10.1016/j.addbeh.2019.01.009

Looby, A., Prince, M.A., Vasko, J.M., Zimmerman, L., Lefler, E.K., Flory, K., Canu, W.H., & Hartung, C.M. (2021). Relations among protective behavioral strategies, biological sex, and ADHD symptoms on alcohol use and related problems: Who benefits most, and from what type of strategy? *Addictive Behaviors.* Advance online publication. 10.1016/j.addbeh.2021.106924

Merkel, R. L., Nichols, J. Q., Fellers, J. C., Hidalgo, P., Martinez, L. A., Putziger, I., Burket, R. C., & Cox, D. J. (2013). Comparison of on-road driving between young adults with and without ADHD. *Journal of Attention Disorders, 20*, 260–269. 10.1177/1087054712473832

Neudecker, C., Mewes, N., Reimers, A.K., & Woll, A. (2019). Exercise Interventions in Children and Adolescents With ADHD: A Systematic Review. *Journal of Attention Disorders*, *23*(4), 307–324. 10.1177/1087054715584053

Nigg, J.T. (2017). *Getting ahead of ADHD: What next-generation science says about treatments that work—and how you can make them work for your child.* Guilford Press.

Rebar, A.L., Stanton, R., Geard, D., Short, C., Duncan, M.J., & Vandelanotte, C. (2015). A meta-meta-analysis of the effect of physical activity on depression and anxiety in non-clinical adult populations. *Health Psychology Review*, *9*(3), 366–378. 10.1080/17437199. 2015.1022901

Richards, T.L., Deffenbacher, J.L., & Rosén, L.A. (2002). Driving anger and other driving-related behaviors in high and low ADHD symptom college students. *Journal of Attention Disorders*, 6(1), 25–3810.1177/108705470200600104

Rooney, M., Chronis-Tuscano, A., & Yoon, Y. (2012). Substance use in college students with ADHD. *Journal of Attention Disorders*, *16*(3), 221–234. 10.1177/1087054710392536

Rooney, M., Chronis-Tuscano, A.M., & Huggins, S. (2015). Disinhibition mediates the relationship between ADHD and problematic alcohol use in college students. *Journal of Attention Disorders*, *19*(4), 313–327. 10.1177/1087054712459885

Rucklidge, J.J., Frampton, C.M., Gorman, B., & Boggis, A. (2017). Vitamin–mineral treatment of ADHD in adults: A 1-year naturalistic follow-up of a randomized controlled trial. *Journal of Attention Disorders*, *21*(6). 522–532. 10.1177/1087054714530557

Serrano, J.W., Abu-Ramadan, T.M., Stevens, A.E., Vasko, J.M., Miller, E., Flory, K., Willcutt, E.G. & Hartung, C.M. (2022). *ADHD and physical exercise in college students: Influence of biological sex.* Unpublished manuscript.

Schulenberg, J.E., Johnston, L.D., O'Malley, P.M., Bachman, J.G., Miech, R.A., & Patrick, M.E. (2020). Monitoring the Future national survey results on drug use, 1975–2019: Volume II, college students and adults ages 19–60. *Institute for Social Research*, University of Michigan.

Sibley, M.H., Swanson, J.M., Arnold, L.E., Hechtman, L.T., Owens, E.B., Stehli, A., Abikoff, H., Hinshaw, S.P., Molina, B., Mitchell, J.T., Jensen, P.S., Howard, A.L., Lakes, K.D., Pelham, W.E., & MTA Cooperative Group (2017). Defining ADHD symptom persistence in adulthood: optimizing sensitivity and specificity. *Journal of Child Psychology And Psychiatry, And Allied Disciplines*, *58*(6), 655–662. 10.1111/jcpp.12620

Taylor, D.J., Bramoweth, A.D., Grieser, E.A., Tatum, J.I., & Roane, B.M. (2013). Epidemiology of insomnia in college students: Relationship with mental health, quality of life, and substance use difficulties. *Behavior Therapy*, *44*(3), 339–348. 10.1016/j.beth. 2012.12.001

Wajszilber, D., Santiseban, J.A., & Gruber, R. (2018). Sleep disorders in patients with ADHD: impact and management challenges. *Nature and Science Of Sleep*, *10*, 453–480. 10.2147/NSS.S163074

Weafer, J., Camarillo, D., Fillmore, M.T., Milich, R., & Marczinski, C.A. (2008). Simulated driving performance of adults with ADHD: comparisons with alcohol intoxication. *Experimental and Clinical Psychopharmacology*, *16*(3), 251–263. 10.1037/ 1064-1297.16.3.251

Werling, A.M., Walitza, S., & Drechsler, R. (2021). Impact of the COVID-19 lockdown on screen media use in patients referred for ADHD to child and adolescent psychiatry: an introduction to problematic use of the internet in ADHD and results of a survey. *Journal of Neural Transmission*, *128*, 1033–1043 10.1007/s00702-021-02332-0

Session 2: Identifying Health-related Behaviors for Goal Setting

Corresponds to Modules 4.1–4.6 in the
Thriving in College Student Workbook

Session Outline

1 Check-in with client(s)
2 Set agenda
3 Review homework
4 Establish and prioritize health-related behavior goals
5 Assess client's motivation for behavior change
6 Discuss homework
7 Schedule the next session

Session Organization

Administration Format

Session 2 should be administered in an individual format since the identification of which behaviors to focus on will be specific to each client. For example, one client may wish to focus only on managing substance use, while another may wish to address all six health-related areas over several individual sessions.

Materials Needed

Attending students should have a notebook or pad of paper or other suitable means (e.g., iPad) to take notes.

Session Content

Check-in with Client(s)

Use this time to solicit brief discussion, or simply to see how things are going and build rapport. Aim for this to be brief (< 5 minutes), encouraging for any additional discussion of this sort to be postponed until after the planned session content is covered. See therapist-client check-in dialogue example in Skill 1: Session 1 as a model for this interaction, if needed. We also recommend having

DOI: 10.4324/9781003149590-20

your client complete the *Progress Tracker* (see Appendix B), and briefly touching base on any declines or improvements in school functioning.

Set Agenda

Introduce the agenda for this session to the client (see Session Outline). It may be helpful to have a visual aid to refer to, such as a flip chart or projected PowerPoint slide or printed handout. At this time it might also be helpful to remind clients to write notes regarding important points in a therapy notebook. Setting the agenda should be speedily completed (< 2 minutes). See therapist-client agenda-setting dialogue example in Skill 1: Session 1 as a model, if needed.

Review Homework from Previous Session

Referring to your notes and the prior module completed, briefly remind the client what their homework assignment was and how you will use that information in this session. Make mental note during this brief activity of any mention of health-related behavior or problems that you may want to make sure are included in subsequent discussion.

Establish and Prioritize Health-related Behavior Goals

In this session, we recommend beginning with a discussion with the client to identify which (if any) of the six areas (i.e., strategies for improving sleep, eating healthier, increasing physical activity, managing substance or technology use, driving safely) the client is interested in addressing and which area they would like to work on first. This discussion will also serve to enhance the client's motivation for making changes in their health-related behaviors. Below is an example dialogue on how to begin (see Dialogue 1) and some suggested prompts for this discussion (see Box 1).

Dialogue 1

Therapist: *In the last session, we talked about how ADHD can impact six areas of physical well-being for college students. We talked about sleep, eating and nutrition, physical activity, substance and technology use, and driving. In today's session, I would like to touch base with you about your current habits in each of these six areas. After we talk about your current habits, then we can discuss whether you would like to make changes in any of these areas at this time. If you choose an area that you would like to work on, then we will identify some goals and strategies for making changes. How does this plan sound to you?*

Client: *It sounds okay. I know I have problems in a couple of these areas but I am not sure if I am ready to make any changes right now. It sounds overwhelming to me. I have struggled with some of these things for a long time.*

Therapist:	*That makes a lot of sense to me. I want you to know that I don't expect you to make any changes right now unless you feel ready. If there are changes you would like to make at this time, I am hoping that with my support, and the skills you have been learning in this program, you might have more success that you've had in the past. Would it be okay with you if we talked through your current habits and then you can let me know if you would like to discuss changes now or hold off until you feel ready?*
Client:	*Yes, that sounds okay.*
Therapist:	*Ok, let's get started by talking about your sleep habits. What time do you usually go to bed?* (Therapist now continues discussion regarding the six health behaviors.)

Box 1 Example prompts for discussion about health-related behaviors

What are your current sleep habits?

- What time do you usually go to bed?
- What time do you usually wake up?
- Do you have trouble falling or staying asleep?
- Do you feel tired during the day?
- How satisfied are you with your current habits?
- Would you like to make a change?
- If so, what kind of change would you like to make?
- If yes, why would you like to make a change (e.g., health, academics, relationships)?
- How confident are you about your ability to make a change in this area at this time?

Describe your current eating habits?

- How many meals per day do you eat?
- How many times per week do you eat out or get take out?
- How many times per week do you cook a healthy meal?
- How satisfied are you with your current habits?
- Would you like to make a change?
- If so, what kind of change would you like to make?
- If yes, why would you like to make a change (e.g., health, academics, relationships)?
- How confident are you about your ability to make a change in this area at this time?

Describe your current physical activity habits?

- How often do you walk or bike for transportation?
- How many times per week do you exercise?
- When you exercise, how long do your workouts usually last?
- What types of activities do you do for exercise?
- How satisfied are you with your current habits?
- Would you like to make a change?
- If so, what kind of change would you like to make (e.g., exercise more or less?)
- If yes, why would you like to make a change (e.g., health, academics, relationships)?
- How confident are you about your ability to make a change in this area at this time?

What are your current substance use habits?

- How many days per week do you use alcohol?
- How many days per week do you use marijuana?
- Do you use any other substances?
- Does drinking alcohol or using marijuana cause any problems for you, like missing class, being hungover, blacking out, or driving under the influence?
- How satisfied are you with your current habits?
- Would you like to make a change?
- If so, what kind of change would you like to make?
- If yes, why would you like to make a change (e.g., health, academics, relationships)?
- How confident are you about your ability to make a change in this area at this time?

What are your current technology use habits?

- How many hours per day do you spend using your "screens" (e.g., texting, gaming, social media, watching TV shows/movies, YouTube, Reddit)?
- Does technology use cause any problems for you (e.g., missing class, getting into arguments online, spending more time or more money using technology than you intended?
- How satisfied are you with your current habits?
- Would you like to make a change?
- If so, what kind of change would you like to make?
- If yes, why would you like to make a change (e.g., health, academics, relationships, finances)?
- How confident are you about your ability to make a change in this area at this time?

What are your current driving habits?

- How often do you drive? What is your driving style like?
- Have you gotten any tickets or citations?
- Do you tend to speed while driving?
- Do you text and drive? Do you change your music or podcast while you are driving?
- Are you often distracted while driving?
- Have you been in any accidents or "near-misses?"
- Do your friends or significant other complain about your driving?
- How satisfied are you with your current habits?
- Would you like to make a change?
- If so, what kind of change would you like to make?
- If yes, why would you like to make a change (e.g., health, legal repercussions, relationships)?
- How confident are you about your ability to make a change in this area at this time?

We include in Appendix A a worksheet (Healthy Lifestyles: Identifying Your Targets) that will help to facilitate this conversation *and* provide a record that can be referred to in the following session.

Assess Client's Motivation for Behavior Change

After identifying the area(s) that the client would like to focus on, the therapist should assess their level of motivation. If a client does not want to make changes in any area but you think that their behaviors in one or more areas might be exacerbating their mental health problems, then you might consider conducting some motivational interviewing at this point (see Dialogue 2).

Dialogue 2

Therapist: *Okay, it sounds like you are fairly satisfied with your eating, physical activity, technology use, and driving habits, but that you might be interested in making some changes with your sleep and alcohol use at some point. For sleep, you said that you would like to get at least 7 hours of sleep per night so that you are better rested and can focus better in your classes. For alcohol use, you said that you wanted to cut back on drinking enough so that you do not ever black out or vomit from drinking. You are worried about the long-term physical effects of drinking so much that these things happen. Does this sound right?*

Client:	*Yes, that's about right. But, I'm really stuck on how to make changes in these areas. I have been trying for a while now but nothing I have tried seems to work. I'm really discouraged by this.*
Therapist:	*I completely understand why you feel discouraged. It can be really hard to make these kinds of lifestyle changes. It sounds like you are a little more confident in your ability to make changes in your sleep habits right now. Would it make sense to you if we started with some sleep changes and held off on the alcohol use changes right now?*
Client:	*Yeah, I am a little more confident about sleep changes so I think it makes sense to start with sleep but I am still worried about my alcohol use.*
Therapist:	*Okay. Let's start with sleep and then, after we see how that goes, we can circle back to alcohol.*
Client:	*That sounds good.*
Therapist:	*Okay. We are about out of time for today. I appreciate your willingness to talk about these lifestyle habits. I know that many of us have struggled in some of these areas for a long time and it can be hard to talk about. Next time we meet, we will talk about some different strategies that other students have found to be helpful in making changes in their sleep habits. I'll help you pick a couple strategies to try and we will talk about using your new OTMP skills to make changes in the areas you have selected.*

Discuss Homework and Schedule Next Session

At this stage, you have guided the client through a fairly thorough consideration of their health-related behaviors, and it should be clear whether they are motivated to pursue any changes in these areas. Still, it's possible that you may need to pose the question: Would you like to change your habits in any of these healthy lifestyle areas? If it is clear that, for your client, the answer is "no," then it may be wise to prioritize another skill in this manual that the client feels more inclined to work on.

It also may be that the assignment of some self-monitoring of behavior (e.g., exercise, eating habits, sleep, technology use) may motivate both those on the fence and those already thinking that they would like to change their behavior into focused action. As such, we generally recommend the assignment of **self-monitoring** (e.g., frequency/intensity of exercise, composition/quantity of meals, quantity of technology use) for a week so that both you and your client(s) understand their baseline for behavior change and can better assess improvement over time. Additionally, you might assign the following question to be completed, based somewhat on the self-monitoring, for next time: What are your goals for improvement in this area (e.g., get 7–9 hours of sleep per night, reduce your alcohol use, exercise three times per week, reduce technology use)?

Session 3: Strategies for Improving Sleep, Eating Healthier, Increasing Physical Activity, Managing Substance and Technology Use, and Driving Safely

Corresponds to Modules 4.1–4.6 in the
Thriving in College Student Workbook

Session Outline

1 Check-in with client(s)
2 Set agenda
3 Review homework
4 Identifying appropriate strategies for health-related behavior change
5 Discuss homework
6 Schedule next session

Session Organization

Administration Format

Session 3 (and subsequent sessions in this skill) should be administered in an individual format since each client will have identified the specific health-related behaviors that they would like to work on. If the student would like to work on several of the six areas, you may need two or more sessions to cover strategies and have the client select which they would like to use.

Materials Needed

You might bring a whiteboard, flipchart, or projected document to capture the ideas of your client or otherwise illustrate important points. Attending students should have a notebook or pad of paper to take notes. It is also advisable to have available copies of the handouts that pertain to the content of this session (see later and Appendix A) to share and/or use with your client(s).

Session Content

Check-in with Client(s)

Use this time to solicit brief discussion, or simply to see how things are going and build rapport. Aim for this to be brief (< 5 minutes), encouraging

DOI: 10.4324/9781003149590-21

for any additional discussion of this sort to be postponed until after the planned session content is covered. See therapist-client check-in dialogue example in Skill 1: Session 1 as a model for this interaction, if needed. We also recommend having your client complete the *Progress Tracker* (see Appendix B), and briefly touching base on any declines or improvements in school functioning.

Set Agenda

Introduce the agenda for this session to the client (see Session Outline). It may be helpful to have a visual aid to refer to, such as a flip chart or projected PowerPoint slide or printed handout. At this time, it might also be helpful to remind clients to write notes regarding important points in a therapy notebook. Setting the agenda should be speedily completed (< 2 minutes). See therapist-client agenda-setting dialogue example in Skill 1: Session 1 as a model, if needed.

Review Homework from Previous Session

Referring to your notes and the prior module completed, briefly remind the client what their homework assignment was and discuss successes and barriers to completion. An aspect of homework that should flow into the content of this session is a focus on the health area(s) or behaviors that were monitored in the last week, and discussion of related goals for change. The introduction of strategies follows from this naturally.

Identifying Appropriate Strategies for Health-related Behavior Change

In this session, we provide numerous ideas for clients to choose from to help them reach their goals in each of these healthy lifestyle areas. Self-determination theory posits that motivation will be improved with a focus on supporting the client's sense of autonomy (Deci & Ryan, 2008). Therefore, we have provided a number of places where clients make choices (e.g., Are you motivated to change in any of these areas? Which area would you like to start with? Which of the strategies I outlined would you like to try first?). We also recommend that therapists discuss the applicability of previously learned OTMP strategies to improving health-related behaviors and have mentioned the use of task lists and calendars in the suggestions given later. Dialogue 1 is an example of how to begin this discussion, here pertaining to sleep.

Dialogue 1

Therapist: *Last week, we identified that you would like to increase your sleep to get at least 7 hours per night so that you feel better rested and can focus better in your classes. Today we are going to review some different strategies that have helped other college students with ADHD improve their sleep habits. The first set of habits are called sleep hygiene habits and they are very helpful for improving the consistency and length of sleep.*

Review the appropriate strategies with your client that are listed here, based on their goals (see example in Dialogue 2); these are also available as handouts in Appendix A.

Sleep: *Which of the following strategies do you use, have you tried, or would you be willing to try to improve your sleep habits?*

- Practice good sleep hygiene habits, which include:
  - Go to bed and wake up at roughly the same time each day, ideally also on weekends (though this is not possible for many college students). It is hard for your brain to adjust to different bedtimes each day.
  - Create a relaxing bedtime routine that does not involve a screen. Ideas include reading a book, listening to music, listening to an audio book, or taking a bath. There are smartphone apps like *Headspace* that include bedtime meditation, and other apps that will read you a bedtime story.
  - Try to stop using screens 30 minutes before bedtime.
  - Make sure your bedroom is cool (between 60 and 67 degrees is ideal).
  - Make sure your bedroom is quiet. Use earplugs or white noise if necessary.
  - Make sure that your bedroom is dark. It is hard to get good sleep with a TV on. Use blackout shades or other window coverings to keep the light out.
  - Finish eating meals 2–3 hours before bedtime. Stop using caffeine 4–6 hours before bedtime.
  - Alcohol and nicotine use can also disrupt sleep. For the best sleep, skip these close to bedtime.
  - Exercise regularly, but don't do vigorous exercise in the evening before bedtime.
  - Sleep on a mattress and pillows that are comfortable and supportive.
  - Don't go to bed unless you are sleepy. And, if you don't fall asleep within 20 minutes of going to bed, get up and do something relaxing.
- Schedule bedtime and wakeup time on your calendar.
- Set multiple alarms to help transition from highly engaging activities to prepare for sleep (e.g., one alarm to turn off screens, one alarm to turn off lights).

- Take your ADHD medications as prescribed. Prescription stimulant medications can disrupt sleep if taken too close to bedtime. Talk to your doctor if your ADHD medication is impacting your sleep.
- Limit your use of sleep aid medication. If you must use a sleep aid medication, melatonin and CBD are both generally safe and typically have no side effects. However, research evidence is limited for both of these sleep aids for insomnia, so it is best to speak with your doctor about options if you believe you need sleep aid medication.
- Seek treatment for co-occurring anxiety and depression as these conditions can also impact sleep in a negative way.
- Track your sleep and how it is impacting behavior. There are wearable devices (e.g., Apple Watch, FitBit) that will track your sleep for you and send the info to a smartphone app.
- Reward yourself for sticking to your new, healthy sleep habits, perhaps with new sheets, comfy PJs or bedroom slippers, or some bubble bath or lotion to use for relaxing before bedtime. Remember your strategies for rewarding yourself from the first few modules of this program.

Dialogue 2

Therapist: *That's a lot of strategies! Are there any of those strategies that you already use or have tried before to improve your sleep?*

Client: *Well, my Apple Watch tells me how long I sleep each night. That's why I know that I only get 5–6 hours of sleep per night. I also know I'm bad about taking a second dose of my Ritalin in the late afternoon or evening when I have a paper to write for my classes or an exam to study for. I also probably use too much Tylenol PM to help me sleep.*

Therapist: *Okay, well it sounds like you have already identified a couple of areas in which you might be able to make some changes. Why don't we write up a plan that you can follow this next week that has some specific strategies from the list given earlier, and also we can come up with some ways to reward yourself for improvements in your sleep duration? It's good you can track that with your Apple Watch.*

Eating: *Which of the following strategies do you use, have you tried, or would you be willing to try?*

- Determine your goals (e.g., eat healthier foods, eat more regularly, reduce emotional eating, lose weight, gain weight, improve blood chemistry).

- Eat several meals per day at regular times so that you have enough energy for your daily activities and do not go so long between meals that you tend to overeat as a result.
- Schedule meals on your calendar if you have difficulty remembering to eat or sticking to a regular eating schedule.
- Plan weekly meals and grocery shop once per week (e.g., Sunday) and schedule this time on your calendar.
- Prepare foods in advance (e.g., make a big pot of soup or a casserole that can be eaten for several meals during the week, prepare fruits and veggies so they can be quickly grabbed, make a big salad) and schedule this on your calendar.
- Prepare meals the night before if you will need to take with you or will not have time during your day (e.g., pack a lunch to take to campus).
- Buy healthy snacks and consider not bringing junk food into the house.
- Put some healthy snacks in your backpack in case you get hungry so that you are not tempted to purchase fast food when you were not planning on it or so that you do not get too hungry and overeat later.
- Keep a food diary or journal or use a smartphone app to track your food intake (e.g., *MyFitnessPal, MyPlate*).
- Plan a certain number of meals per week that you will eat out or get takeout and stick to your plans.
- Get familiar with recommended nutrition guidelines or visit a nutritionist if your student health service has one available.
- Buy a cookbook or subscribe to a recipe or meal planning site (e.g., Cooking Light, NYT Cooking).

Physical activity: *Which of the following strategies do you use, have you tried, or would you be willing to try?*

- Transportation
  - Walk or bike to work or on errands if feasible.
  - Take the stairs instead of the elevator.
  - Park further away from the store on purpose.
  - Use an activity or step tracker (e.g., FitBit, Garmin watch, Apple watch) with a smartphone app and set a daily steps goal.

- Exercise
  - Set a goal for how many times per week you would like to exercise. Let clients choose whether they want to focus on further, longer or faster.
  - Put exercise on your calendar and build into your day.
  - Consider whether you prefer working out alone or with others.

- Find an accountability or work-out partner (e.g., make plans to workout with a friend to increase the likelihood that you will follow through). If your friend is at a different skill level, you could have a plan to go together but not exercise together (e.g., swim at different speeds).
- Consider joining a yoga studio or a gym. This can be helpful if you do not have a reliable workout partner because you might develop acquaintances or friendships at the gym and you might look forward to seeing these folks. You might also be more likely to go to an exercise class if you have already paid for it in advance.
- Pick physical activities that you enjoy doing or that you find less aversive (e.g., if you dislike running because of the physical challenge, start with walking). Listen to music or an audiobook while exercising to make the experience more pleasant. Some researchers have referred to this as "temptation bundling" (e.g., Kirgios et al., 2020) and suggest only allowing yourself to listen to a particularly compelling book while exercising.
- Join a club or a class to learn a new activity (e.g., take an introduction to cross-country skiing at outdoor program, attend a group workout class at campus recreation center).
- Schedule exercise more frequently to plan for the inevitable times when it doesn't work out due to other more urgent tasks (e.g., if you want to exercise 3 times per week, then schedule 5 times knowing that you can skip 2 if the timing isn't working out).
- Use a smartphone app that allows you to see what your friends and acquaintances are doing (e.g., Strava).
- Reward yourself for meeting your daily steps goal or increasing your exercise sessions, perhaps with a new work-out outfit, tennis shoes, or a healthy smoothie.

Substance use: *Which of the following strategies do you use, have you tried, or would you be willing to try?*

- Track your use of alcohol and drugs. Set a goal of reducing use. Reward yourself for progress in this area, perhaps with a fun activity with friends that does not involve drinking or using drugs like playing paintball, going out for coffee, or taking a walk.
- There are several protective behavioral strategies that have been shown through research to be helpful to college students with ADHD for reducing alcohol use and the negative outcomes associated with use such as blacking out, being hungover, driving drunk, and missing class. Select the strategies that you think will be most helpful for you from the following list.

○ Set a limit on the number of drinks you will have in one drinking session. If you don't think you can keep track, put that many rubber bands on one wrist and each time you have a drink, remove a rubber band and put it in your pocket.

○ Mix and bring your own beverages. When what you bought is gone, stop drinking.

○ Avoid combining alcohol and marijuana. Combining substances can make you get more drunk/high and reduce your ability to make good decisions about limiting your use and staying safe.

○ Avoid pre-gaming or pre-partying.

○ Stop drinking at a predetermined time and drink water only after this time. This will also help you sleep better.

○ Eat a meal before or during drinking.

○ Avoid mixing different types of alcohol.

○ Drink slowly rather than gulping or chugging. If you feel pressure to drink more, you can always pretend to take a sip now and then. You can also take your drink to the kitchen or bathroom or outside and pour some out.

○ Avoid trying to keep up or out drink others. Avoid drinking games.

○ Alternate alcoholic and nonalcoholic drinks. For every alcoholic drink you have, drink a glass of water. Or, put extra ice in your alcoholic drink to water it down.

○ Ask a friend to let you know when you have had enough to drink.

○ Only go out with people you know and trust and make sure you are with people who can take care of you if you drink too much.

○ Know where your drink has been at all times. Keep it in your hand. If you are at a party, bring your own drink container with a lid. These strategies will help to prevent others from "drugging" your drink.

○ Use a designated driver or a ride service like Uber.

Technology Use: *Which of the following strategies do you use, have you tried, or would you be willing to try?*

• Use airplane mode on your phone or turn off the internet on your computer to limit distractions when you are trying to be productive.

• Track your screen time using the settings on your phone or an app. Set a goal of reducing use. Reward yourself for progress in this area, perhaps with a fun activity with friends that does not involve technology like playing baseball, going out for coffee, or taking a walk.

• Set a limit on the number of minutes or hours you will spend per day engaging in a particular type of technology use (e.g., video gaming). Use phone timers or apps to remind yourself.

- Ask your partner, friend, or roommate to set shared goals regarding technology use (e.g., video gaming, Netflix) and try to hold each other accountable.
- Put your phone in the middle of the table when you are at a restaurant and ask your dining partners to do the same. You can make a game out of it by saying that whoever checks their phone first must pay the bill.
- Make a point of putting your phone in another room or in a location where you cannot easily access it (e.g., a drawer) while you are doing schoolwork or spending time with friends or use an app that doesn't allow you to use it while you are doing a pomodoro (e.g., Forest or Flora).
- Carry a book with you so that you can read instead of watching YouTube or checking social media when you have a little down time between activities or must wait for a class or appointment.
- Use technology as a reward for completing other activities (e.g., when I finish this assignment, I will use my phone for 5 minutes; when I finish all my homework, I will play video games for an hour).

Driving Safely: *Which of the following strategies do you use, have you tried, or would you be willing to try?*

- If you take stimulant medicine for your ADHD, take it regularly at the scheduled time. You will be a more attentive driver if you are taking your medication as prescribed. Obviously, driving does not happen just on weekdays!
- Schedule long driving trips early in the day when you are rested and alert. Take a break every 2 hours.
- Set your phone to automatically go to do-not-disturb when you are driving. Leave your phone in the backseat or trunk while you are driving.
- Adjust your radio or look up driving directions before you begin a drive, not during the drive.
- Limit the number of passengers that you take in your car to reduce distractions while driving (e.g., driving 5 drunk friends to a party may be very distracting).
- Make a commitment not to drive after drinking or using drugs.
- Consider taking a taxi, Uber, or Lyft instead of driving if there is a large group or anyone has been drinking or using drugs (if these services are not available where you are, call a friend).

Discuss Homework and Schedule Next Session

Ask your client, for the healthy lifestyle area(s) they have chosen to work on first, to select a few strategies to try this week; make sure your client has written these down along with some detail of how to implement them. Instruct your client to track their use of these strategies, much as they used self-monitoring of their behavior in the previous week's homework.

References

Deci, E.L., & Ryan, R.M. (2008). Self-determination theory: A macrotheory of human motivation, development, and health. *Canadian Psychology/Psychologie canadienne, 49*(3), 182–185. 10.1037/a0012801

Kirgios, E.L., Mandel, G.H., Park, Y., Milkman, K.L., Gromet, D.M., Kay, J.S., & Duckworth, A.L. (2020). Teaching temptation bundling to boost exercise: A field experiment. *Organizational Behavior and Human Decision Processes, 161*, 20–25. 10.1016/j.obhdp.2020.09.003

Skill 5: Being Successful in Relationships

(~3 sessions)

Corresponds to Skillset 5 of the *Thriving in College* Student Workbook

Background for the Therapist

In general, research suggests that when we have stable and satisfying relationships we tend to be better adjusted in life (e.g., Eakin et al., 2004; Musick & Bumpass, 2012). One of things that you may already know or appreciate even from what has been covered elsewhere in this manual is that ADHD is associated with characteristics that can pose problems in social relationships, in childhood, adolescence, and adulthood. Approximately 50% of children with ADHD (Hoza et al., 2005) experience widespread peer rejection. Their impulsive and inattentive behaviors, such as not following the rules of a game, acting out of turn, or using inappropriate play behaviors (e.g., disruptive interruptions), can very quickly cause other children to withdraw from interactions and to begin disliking them (Milich & Landau, 1982; Ronk et al., 2011), which can be thought of as the leading edge of social rejection. In their elementary school classrooms, children with ADHD exhibit more disruptive behaviors, and also have lower ability to withstand provocation by peers to act out (Frankel & Feinberg, 2002). As these experiences pile up, children with ADHD develop a negative social reputation in their peer groups (Erhardt & Hinshaw, 1994), which becomes very difficult for them to overcome. Friendships, defined by mutually satisfying interactions and support that is not limited to in-school experience, are much less common in this group of socially rejected children with ADHD than in peers without ADHD (Hoza, 2007). When friendships do exist, they tend to be characterized by relative instability, lower cooperation and support, and higher conflict, and neutral observers rate the behavior of the children with ADHD as being more self-centered, insensitive, and rule-breaking (Mikami, 2010; Normand et al., 2011, 2019). Friendships tend to be with other children on the margins of the "socially-accepted" group. Unfortunately for the children with ADHD, such peers may also tend toward disruptive, oppositional, or even delinquent behaviors, which provides no modeling of positive and adaptive behaviors that could assist the child or adolescent with ADHD to change their social status (Hoza et al., 2005;

DOI: 10.4324/9781003149590-22

Marshall et al., 2014; Murray-Close et al., 2010; Normand et al., 2011). In addition, children with ADHD often fail to observe their own social blunders, a phenomenon that has been called the positive illusory bias, which prevents them from actively focusing on implementing new, more adaptive behaviors (Hoza, 2007). Children with maladjustment in this domain are at high risk for negative outcomes in school and, later, in work, criminal behaviors, and psychiatric hospitalization, among others (Milich & Landau, 1982), so peer relationship problems may have pervasive impact. Thus, college students with ADHD may have a long history of problematic peer relationships that in turn influence their current social behaviors, adjustment, and self-regard.

Unfortunately, social adjustment for children with ADHD can even be problematic in their own families. While there may be some differences between families based on the specific presentation of ADHD (i.e., with or without hyperactivity) and presence of comorbid disruptive behaviors, a seminal review paper by Johnston and Mash (2001) outlines how families of children with ADHD are characterized by high stress and conflict and more frequent negative parenting behaviors (e.g., authoritarian/punitive and/or permissive parenting), which may be exacerbated by comorbid oppositional or conduct disorder (Deault, 2010). Parents (with mothers being most studied) have been observed to interact more negatively and less socially with their children with ADHD, and to be more demanding. Mothers report disagreements with their children with ADHD occurring five times more often than do mothers with neurotypical children, and anger arises in those interactions seven times more often (Whalen et al., 2006). As a result, parental relationships for colleges students with ADHD may include a long history of strife that may take some work to resolve.

While the peer relationships of adolescents with ADHD are less well studied than those in childhood, existent research suggest that, for many, social-behavioral deficits and peer rejection persist (Owens et al., 2009). Importantly, poor social acceptance (as well as inattentive symptoms) in early adolescence has been shown to be predictive of poorer academic outcomes in junior high and high school (Dvorsky et al., 2018). Further, in this period of increased child drive for independence, conflict and negative feelings in parent-child relationships seems to persist and appears to be most severe in families with a child with ADHD. Conflict may be evoked by the child's disruptive or off-task behavior. Compellingly, in college students with ADHD, a negative parent-child relationship can be exacerbated by high levels of achievement orientation in the family (Grenwald-Mayes, 2002), one of the very things that might motivate an adolescent with ADHD to continue their education.

New and developmentally important romantic relationships emerge in adolescence, too, and differences have been noted in the timing and characteristics of such relationships in those with and without ADHD. Consistently, adolescents and emerging adults with ADHD tend toward earlier sex (especially in males and teens with prominent hyperactivity-impulsivity), more numerous sexual partners (see exception, for women, in Babinski et al., 2011) and truncated relationships (Rokeach & Wiener, 2018). Men with the inattentive presentation of ADHD, at least in emerging adulthood, may buck this trend, in that they appear to be less romantically active and are viewed as less desirable partners by same-age women (Canu & Carlson, 2003). In general, the relationships of adolescents and adults with ADHD may have lower rates of intimacy (Ben-Naim et al., 2017; Margherio et al., 2021; Marsh et al., 2015), and those who are sexually active are more likely to engage in unprotected sex and to suffer related consequences (e.g., sexually transmitted disease, unplanned pregnancy; Flory et al., 2006). As such, college students with ADHD may need support to develop healthy relationships and navigate the risks and rewards of intimacy.

Conflict resolution styles have also been shown to differ in emerging adult couples with an ADHD partner, with higher rates of negative, aversive behaviors that can have a deleterious effect on relational satisfaction (Canu & Carlson, 2007; Canu et al., 2014). Further, college students with elevated ADHD symptoms tend to experience higher degrees of anger, which could have a toxic effect in relationships (Sacchetti & Lefler, 2017). At its extreme, the romantic relationships of those with ADHD are marked by higher rates of verbal and physical aggression (Fang et al., 2010; Wymbs et al., 2012), and such victimization unfortunately seems to extend to sexual victimization (White & Buehler, 2012). It is important to note that not all couples with an ADHD partner feature all or even any of these characteristics, but it is important to be alert to the myriad of risk factors for adjustment in adult romantic relationships (for review, see Wymbs et al., 2021). It is also important to note that most of these findings are based on largely white, heterosexual samples, and thus it is unclear how much they generalize to the relationships of the LBGTQ+, gender queer, and/or non-white populations with ADHD.

Just as most people do not "outgrow" their ADHD symptoms, relationship problems often continue for people with ADHD into adulthood. Adults with ADHD report less satisfaction in their family and social lives (Biederman et al., 2006), and the emotional dysregulation that often co-occurs with the disorder is related to higher degrees of conflict, hostile behavior, and lower romantic relational quality (Bruner et al., 2015) that could account for more frequent divorce and separation (Biederman et al., 2006). Spouses of people with ADHD identify specific behaviors that are most difficult and make them feel unloved such including both inattentive behavior (not remembering things they are told, zoning out in conversations) and impulsive behavior (saying things without thinking). Notably, behavior of women with ADHD may be rated by their husbands as more aversive than that of men with ADHD by their wives (Robin & Payson, 2002). Emerging adults with ADHD have also been shown to have difficulty providing effective emotional support to and managing conflict in their friendships, but the effects of ADHD on relationship quality appears to be mitigated if the level of ADHD symptoms between friends is similar (McKee, 2017).

Family members of emerging adults with ADHD tend to see their relationships as problematic and the behavior of their loved one with ADHD being more hostile, but this may often escape the notice of the family member with ADHD (similar to the positive illusory bias noted in childhood; Sodano et al., 2019), which likely only adds to relational distancing.

While research on social outcomes in emerging adults with ADHD remains sparse, this body of evidence suggests that many college students with ADHD may have encountered peer rejection, parent-child relational problems, and other forms of social maladjustment, and may continue to experience these problems during the college years. Social problems may impact success in relationships in work, and necessary interactions with others in school, too. Although social adjustment at work has not been a substantive area of empirical research, it is clear that adults with ADHD tend to underperform in the workplace and have difficulty finding a career track that suits their needs.

The sessions in this module provide a starting point to helping clients address the social problems they may be encountering. As with other skills, some clients may need no remediation in this area. Others may only need to focus on one area (e.g., romantic relationships). If it is clear that relationships and/or work adjustment are areas of concern for your client(s), then the best starting point is Session 1 (Psychoeducation), which will set up an informed discussion about which other sessions are appropriate.

Student Workbook

If you are using the *Thriving in College* student workbook, you will find that Skillset 5 on *Building Strong Relationships* corresponds to the material in this section. The chart below provides more information on which individual modules in the workbook correspond to each session in this section.

Therapist Guide Session	Workbook Modules
1	5.0 Why it Matters, Pre-Assessment, & Roadmap
2	5.1 Improve Relationships with Friends and Partners
3	5.2 Navigate Your Relationship with Your Parents

References

Babinski, D.E., Pelham, W.E., Jr, Molina, B.S., Gnagy, E.M., Waschbusch, D.A., Yu, J., Maclean, M.G., Wymbs, B.T., Sibley, M.H., Biswas, A., Robb, J.A., & Karch, K.M. (2011). Late adolescent and young adult outcomes of girls diagnosed with ADHD in childhood: An exploratory investigation. *Journal of Attention Disorders, 15*(3), 204–214. 10.1177/1087054710361586

Biederman, J., Faraone, S.V., Spencer, T.J., Mick, E., Monuteaux, M.C., & Aleardi, M. (2006). Functional impairments in adults with self-reports of diagnosed ADHD: A controlled study of 1001 adults in the community. *The Journal of Clinical Psychiatry, 67*(4), 524–540. 10.4088/jcp.v67n0403

Ben-Naim, S., Marom, I., Krashin, M., Gifter, B., & Arad, K. (2017). Life with a partner with ADHD: The moderating role of intimacy. *Journal of Child and Family Studies, 26*, 1365–1373. 10.1007/S10826-016-0653-9

Bruner, M.R., Kuryluk, A.D., & Whitton, S.W. (2015). Attention-deficit/hyperactivity disorder symptom levels and romantic relationship quality in college students. *Journal of American College Health, 63*(2), 98–108. 10.1080/07448481.2014.975717

Canu, W.H., & Carlson, C.L. (2003). Differences in heterosocial behavior and outcomes of ADHD-symptomatic subtypes in a college sample. *Journal of Attention Disorders, 6*(3), 123–133. 10.1177/108705470300600304

Canu, W.H., & Carlson, C.L. (2007). Rejection sensitivity and social outcomes of young adult men with ADHD. *Journal of Attention Disorders, 10*(3), 261–275. 10.1177/1087054 706288106

Canu, W.H., Tabor, L.S., Michael, K.D., Bazzini, D.G., & Elmore, A.L. (2014). Young adult romantic couples' conflict resolution and satisfaction varies with partner's attention-deficit/hyperactivity disorder type. *Journal of Marital and Family Therapy, 40*(4), 509–524. 10.1111/jmft.12018

Deault L.C. (2010). A systematic review of parenting in relation to the development of comorbidities and functional impairments in children with attention-deficit/ hyperactivity disorder (ADHD). *Child Psychiatry and Human Development, 41*(2), 168–192. 10.1007/s10578-009-0159-4

Dvorsky, M.R., Langberg, J.M., Evans, S.W., & Becker, S.P. (2018). The protective effects of social factors on the academic functioning of adolescents With ADHD. *Journal of Clinical Child and Adolescent Psychology: The Official Journal for the Society of Clinical Child and Adolescent Psychology, American Psychological Association, Division 53, 47*(5), 713–726. 10.1080/15374416.2016.1138406

Eakin, L., Minde, K., Hechtman, L., Ochs, E., Krane, E., Bouffard, R., Greenfield, B., & Looper, K. (2004). The marital and family functioning of adults with ADHD and their spouses. *Journal of Attention Disorders, 8*(1), 1–10. 10.1177/108705470400800101

Erhardt, D., & Hinshaw, S.P. (1994). Initial sociometric impressions of attention-deficit hyperactivity disorder and comparison boys: Predictions from social behaviors and from nonbehavioral variables. *Journal of Consulting and Clinical Psychology, 62*(4), 833–842. 10.1037/0022-006X.62.4.833

Fang, X., Massetti, G.M., Ouyang, L., Grosse, S.D., & Mercy, J.A. (2010). Attention-deficit/hyperactivity disorder, conduct disorder, and young adult intimate partner violence. *Archives of General Psychiatry, 67*(11), 1179–1186. 10.1001/archgenpsychiatry. 2010.137

Flory, K., Molina, B.S., Pelham, W.E., Jr, Gnagy, E., & Smith, B. (2006). Childhood ADHD predicts risky sexual behavior in young adulthood. *Journal of Clinical Child and aDolescent Psychology: tHe Official Journal for the Society of Clinical Child and Adolescent Psychology, American Psychological Association, Division 53, 35*(4), 571–577. 10.1207/s153 74424jccp3504_8

Frankel, F., & Feinberg, D. (2002). Social problems associated with ADHD vs. ODD in children referred for friendship problems. *Child Psychiatry and Human Development, 33*(2), 125–146. 10.1023/A:1020730224907

Grenwald-Mayes, G. (2002). Relationship between current quality of life and family of origin dynamics for college students with Attention-Deficit/Hyperactivity Disorder. *Journal of Attention Disorders, 5*(4), 211–222. 10.1177/108705470100500403

Hoza B. (2007). Peer functioning in children with ADHD. *Ambulatory Pediatrics: The Official Journal of the Ambulatory Pediatric Association, 7*(1 Suppl), 101–106. 10.1016/j.ambp.2006.04.011

Hoza, B., Mrug, S., Gerdes, A.C., Hinshaw, S.P., Bukowski, W.M., Gold, J.A., Kraemer, H.C., Pelham, W.E., Jr, Wigal, T., & Arnold, L.E. (2005). What aspects of peer relationships are impaired in children with attention-deficit/hyperactivity disorder?. *Journal of Consulting and Clinical Psychology, 73*(3), 411–423. 10.1037/0022-006X.73.3.411

Johnston, C., & Mash, E.J. (2001). Families of children with Attention-Deficit/Hyperactivity Disorder: Review and recommendations for future research. *Clinical Child and Family Psychology Review, 4*(3), 183–207. 10.1023/A:1017592030434

Margherio, S.M., Capps, E.R., Monopoli, J.W., Evans, S.W., Hernandez-Rodriguez, M., Owens, J.S., & DuPaul, G.J. (2021). Romantic relationships and sexual behavior among adolescents with ADHD. *Journal of Attention Disorders, 25*(10), 1466–1478. 10.1177/1087054720914371

Marsh, L.E., Norvilitis, J.M., Ingersoll, T.S., & Li, B. (2015). ADHD symptomatology, fear of intimacy, and sexual anxiety and behavior among college students in China and the United States. *Journal of Attention Disorders, 19*(3), 211–221. 10.1177/1087054712453483

Marshall, S.A., Evans, S.W., Eiraldi, R.B., Becker, S.P., & Power, T.J. (2014). Social and academic impairment in youth with ADHD, predominantly inattentive type and sluggish cognitive tempo. *Journal of Abnormal Child Psychology, 42*(1), 77–90. 10.1007/s10802-013-9758-4

McKee T.E. (2017). Peer relationships in undergraduates With ADHD Symptomatology: Selection and quality of friendships. *Journal of aTtention Disorders, 21*(12), 1020–1029. 10.1177/1087054714554934

Mikami A.Y. (2010). The importance of friendship for youth with attention-deficit/hyperactivity disorder. *Clinical Child and Family Psychology Review, 13*(2), 181–198. 10.1007/s10567-010-0067-y

Milich, R., & Landau, S. (1982). Socialization and peer relations in hyperactive children. In K.D. Gadow & I. Bialer. (Eds.), *Advances in learning and behavioral disabilities* (Vol. 1, pp283–339). JAI Press.

Murray-Close, D., Hoza, B., Hinshaw, S.P., Arnold, L.E., Swanson, J., Jensen, P.S., Hechtman, L., & Wells, K. (2010). Developmental processes in peer problems of children with attention-deficit/hyperactivity disorder in the Multimodal Treatment Study of Children With ADHD: Developmental cascades and vicious cycles. *Development and psychopathology, 22*(4), 785–802. 10.1017/S0954579410000465

Musick, K. & Bumpass, L. (2012). Reexamining the case for marriage: Union formation and changes in well-being. *Journal of Marriage and Family 74*(1), 1–18. 10.1111/j.1741-3737.2011.00873.x

Normand, S., Schneider, B.H., Lee, M.D., Maisonneuve, M.F., Kuehn, S.M., & Robaey, P. (2011). How do children with ADHD (mis)manage their real-life dyadic friendships? A multi-method investigation. *Journal of Abnormal Child Psychology, 39*(2), 293–305. 10.1007/s10802-010-9450-x

Normand, S., Soucisse, M.M., Melançon, M., Schneider, B.H., Lee, M.D., & Maisonneuve, M.F. (2019). Observed free-play patterns of children with ADHD and their real-life friends. *Journal of Abnormal Child Psychology, 47*(2), 259–271. 10.1007/s10802-018-0437-3

Owens, E.B., Hinshaw, S.P., Lee, S.S., & Lahey, B.B. (2009). Few girls with childhood attention-deficit/hyperactivity disorder show positive adjustment during adolescence. *Journal of Clinical Child and Adolescent Psychology, 38*(1), 132–143. 10.1080/1537441 0802575313

Robin, A.L., & Payson, E. (2002). The impact of ADHD on marriage. *The ADHD Report, 10*, 9–14. https://doi.org/abs101521adhd103920553

Rokeach, A., & Wiener, J. (2018). The romantic relationships of adolescents with ADHD. *Journal of Attention Disorders, 22*(1), 35–45. 10.1177/1087054714538660

Ronk, M.J., Hund, A.M., & Landau, S. (2011). Assessment of social competence of boys with attention-deficit/hyperactivity disorder: Problematic peer entry, host responses, and evaluations. *Journal of Abnormal Child Psychology, 39*(6), 829–840. 10.1007/s10802-011-9497-3

Sacchetti, G.M., & Lefler, E.K. (2017). ADHD symptomology and social functioning in college students. *Journal of Attention Disorders, 21*(12), 1009–1019. 10.1177/1087054 714557355

Sodano, S.M., Tamulonis, J.P., Fabiano, G.A., Caserta, A.M., Hulme, K.F., Hulme, K.L., Stephan, G.R., & Tronci, F. (2019). Interpersonal problems of young adults with and without attention-deficit/hyperactivity disorder. *Journal of Attention Disorders, 25*(4), 562–571. 10.1177/1087054718821728

Whalen, C.K., Henker, B., Ishikawa, S.S., Jamner, L.D., Floro, J.N., Johnston, J.A., & Swindle, R. (2006). An electronic diary study of contextual triggers and ADHD: Get ready, get set, get mad. *Journal of the American Academy of Child and Adolescent Psychiatry, 45*(2), 166–174. 10.1097/01.chi.0000189057.67902.10

White, J.W., & Buehler, C. (2012). Adolescent sexual victimization, ADHD symptoms, and risky sexual behavior. *Journal of Family Violence, 27*(2), 123–132. 10.1007/s10896-012-9411-y

Wymbs, B. T., Canu, W. H., Sacchetti, G. M., & Ranson, L. M. (2021). Adult ADHD and romantic relationships: What we know and what we can do to help. *Journal of Marital and Family Therapy, 47*(3), 664–681. 10.1111/jmft.12475

Wymbs, B., Molina, B., Pelham, W., Cheong, J., Gnagy, E., Belendiuk, K., Walther, C., Babinski, D., & Waschbusch, D. (2012). Risk of intimate partner violence among young adult males with childhood ADHD. *Journal of Attention Disorders, 16*(5), 373–383. 10.1177/1087054710389987

Session 1: Learning about Relationships, Relationship Skills, and ADHD

Corresponds to Module 5.0 of the *Thriving in College* Student Workbook

Session Outline

1 Check-in with client(s)
2 Set agenda
3 Discuss trends in relationships for people with ADHD
4 Discuss aspects of effective communication
5 Discuss homework
6 Schedule next session

Session Organization

Administration Format

Session 1 can be administered in a group or individual format. A group session may be optimal in that the presence of other students with ADHD may validate some of the shared experiences about relationships. However, the session can also be efficiently and effectively employed for an individual client, if a group format is not practical.

Materials Needed

The therapist should have a whiteboard, flipchart, or a projected digital document to capture group ideas and/or present material.

- A list or handout with "take home messages" regarding the session's content as well as instructions/goals for at-home work prior to the next session is also helpful.
- In addition, worksheets (see examples below) that facilitate awareness of relational history and forms (see below) that help clients to learn about their own communication style, for use in session and as homework

As always, therapists are reminded to instruct clients ahead of the session to bring a notebook or device in which they can take notes.

DOI: 10.4324/9781003149590-23

Session Content

Check-in with Client(s)

It is unlikely that this will be the first technique or content-heavy session that a client has done with you. Check-in time can be used to solicit brief discussion about homework or issues that the client is dealing with currently, or simply to see how things are going and strengthen rapport. In the event that this session is the first meeting with clients, check-in might focus more on feelings and expectations about therapy. In any event, aim for this to be brief (< 5 minutes), encouraging client(s) to postpone any additional discussion of this sort until after the session content is completed. See therapist-client check-in dialogue example in Skill 1: Session 1 as a model for this interaction, if needed. We also recommend having your client complete the Progress Tracker (see Appendix B), and briefly touching base on any declines or improvements in school functioning.

Set Agenda

Introduce the agenda for this session to the client (see Session Outline). It is helpful to have a visual aid to refer to, such as a flip chart or projected PowerPoint slide or printed handout. At this time it might also be helpful to remind clients to write notes regarding important points in a therapy notebook. Setting the agenda should be speedily completed (< 2 minutes). See therapist-client agenda-setting dialogue example in Skill 1: Session 1 as a model, if needed.

Discuss Trends in Relationships for People with ADHD

Begin by opening a dialogue about how the client perceives their own experiences in relationships. If extensive information is already available (e.g., discovered in clinical intake interview), then this can more take the form of an informed review and factual check in about what you know (e.g., had real difficulty in keeping friends in childhood, has had meaningful romantic relationships but also struggled in them). See Dialogue 1 for an example discussion with a cisgendered, heterosexual male college student.

Dialogue 1 Example dialogue with a cis-gendered heterosexual man

Therapist: *I'd like to start today by just talking about what it's been like for you in your relationships, in the past and today. Have you found it to be easy, or hard sometimes or in some ways?*

Client: *Sure … so, do you mean like in friendships, or romantic relationships, or just with people in general?*

Therapist:	*Actually, all of that would be good to consider, yes.*
Client:	*Oh, OK. I suppose that it's a mix of easy and hard ... maybe harder than easy, now that I think about it. I've never considered myself someone who has a hard time meeting others, it's kind of the opposite because I'm pretty outgoing. I guess I have trouble making real friends, though. Sometimes I think someone is my friend but then find out they really could care less about me ... I guess that happened a lot when I was a kid. I had a few friends who were good, but mostly I didn't get along great with other kids. I also had a hard time with my parents, to be honest ... sometimes I didn't really feel that close with them, they were angry with me a lot and said they worried about me or were frustrated by things I did.*
Therapist:	*It sounds like you have experienced your fair share of rejection, there.*
Client:	*Yeah. Sometimes things got pretty lonely for me. Then something would happen and I would have a friend or two and it would be OK. That was easiest actually when my family moved.*
Therapist:	*Kind of like a blank slate, I guess?*
Client:	*That's a good way to put it. Over time, I also began to know my place. It seemed like I could never really get along with the kids who were popular or were super-serious about school, but there were some other kids that didn't really care how I acted, who were kind of "outsiders" themselves.*
Therapist:	*I see. Sounds like with those kids, for better or worse, there was some common ground.*
Client:	*Yep. I remember some would think it was cool that I would just blurt out things and interrupt what was going on in class or fluster the teacher. I mostly didn't mean to do it, but some of my friends not only tolerated it but liked it.*
Therapist:	*So, you said that you and your parents didn't have the closest relationship?*
Client:	*As a kid, well, as a teenager, too, that was definitely the case. Or, at least that's the way it felt. I kind of knew deep down that they loved me, but we also were constantly bickering, and sometimes it just felt like they were taskmasters. Now that I've been away from home for a little bit, I appreciate them a little more ... in fact, our relationship has gotten a little better, especially when I'm away at school.*
Therapist:	*So, does that mean that there is conflict between you and them when you go back home?*
Client:	*Well ... yeah ... not as bad as it was, but they still get all into my business. I feel like they don't trust me to do the right thing, to be able to live my life and be a success.*
Therapist:	*I get that. I think a lot of college students feel that way ... do you think it's different because you have ADHD?*

Client:	*I think so. Like I said, I appreciate all the things that they did to help me when I was in high school, you know, like helping remind me about stuff and also making sure I had a good place to study and that sort of thing. But I think they helped me a lot more than my other friends' parents did. I think that they kind of have a hard time letting go of that, especially when I'm home.*
Therapist:	*Yeah. I guess that makes some sense.*
Client:	*I guess so!*
Therapist:	*So, you haven't hit on romantic relationships. What have those been like for you?*
Client:	*That's ... well, now that I think about it, it's kind of been like with my friendships. I started dating, I mean like hanging out with girls I liked when I was pretty young, like 12 or 13. Again, they were mostly like me ... kinda fringe ... didn't mind taking risks sometimes. But it wasn't easy as a kid, it was confusing sometimes, like I didn't know what I wanted or what they wanted or how to act, and relationships kinda came and went, all through high school. In college, I've hung out with women and messed around and stuff but I haven't really had a good, long relationship yet.*
Therapist:	*In all this, would you say that you've been happy?*
Client:	*It's weird, sometimes yeah pretty happy, like I thought things were going really well ... but then I'd find out the hard way that things really weren't going well, like someone would just kind of leave me cold.*
Therapist:	*That hurts when that happens.*
Client:	*Heck yeah it does. Sometimes I just had no idea why, and that makes it even worse.*
Therapist:	*Well, hopefully what we'll talk about and work on in the next several sessions is going to help make that sort of thing happen less often in your life.*
Client:	*I would really like that, yeah!*

At this point, it is likely, as in this example, that the client will have hit on several of their own experiences that mirror what the research suggests is common for kids and/or teens with ADHD. These should serve as springboards for you to introduce these common trends and provide structure for the discussion about trends in relationships with ADHD. Relate their experiences to matching (or contrasting) psychoeducational detail (see the material for the therapist at the beginning of this skill). Lead-in statements and matching topics to highlight might include (**but are not limited to**) things like:

- *You mentioned having difficulty making and keeping friends. That's something that is really quite common for kids with ADHD ... .* discuss how around half of children with

ADHD experience peer rejection, how certain behaviors like rule-breaking lead to negative impressions, how negative social status can be "sticky" across grades, how it's not really about ignorance of social skills but inability to use them when needed.

- *You said that you and your parents didn't really see eye to eye and that you didn't have a close relationship with them. There's a lot that could go into that, for anyone, but for kids with ADHD* ... discuss how parent-child relationships can often be strained when a child has ADHD, how interactions tend to have more of a negative tinge to them, how emotions like anger are more common, how emotional dysregulation of ADHD is involved, how the common parent "playbook" doesn't work for kids with ADHD, how kids with ADHD tend to need more salient and immediate rewards for "good" behavior to learn and how parents often don't know that.

- *I'm hearing you say that* [your current and/or past] *romantic relationships have been kind of rocky, that you haven't been totally happy in them. While that's really not that unusual for adolescents and young adults, research has documented that this can be more of thing for people with ADHD than for others* ... discuss how for many with ADHD they may start "dating" substantially earlier than peers without ADHD, and how that may be difficult to navigate ... discuss how emotional dysregulation related to ADHD and executive dysfunction can contribute to more intensely experienced anger in relationships ... discuss how ADHD is associated with potentially problematic decisions, like unsafe sex ... discuss how ADHD maps onto negative conflict resolution styles ... discuss how certain inattentive and/or impulsive behaviors can aggravate partners, when untreated.

It is important in this discussion to be empathic, encouraging, *and* realistic. ADHD has in general been shown to predict social difficulties, as reviewed above. Clients will likely be receptive to a brief review of the sorts of findings that support this trend, but it may be most helpful to couch this information in ways that emphasize that they are not alone in this (i.e., many others with ADHD have a hard time, too) and that they do face some natural hurdles that others do not. This may be something that is easy to do in a group format, as there will be opportunities for clients to share their experiences; if you are seeing a client individually and using this session, you may want to come prepared with specific examples of relational difficulties to describe to "join with" your client (e.g., Robin and Payson (2002) describe things that are "most aggravating" for partners of adults with ADHD, see Box 1). At the same time, it is also important to bolster their motivation for change, emphasizing that knowing these common pitfalls and especially recognizing which are most problematic for the client will lead to knowing what can be changed for the better.

Box 1   Most frequently endorsed behaviors that make partners of people with ADHD feel unloved, unimportant, and ignored (Robin & Payson, 2002)

1 Doesn't remember being told things
2 Leaves a mess
3 Doesn't finish household projects
4 Zones out in conversations
5 Says things without thinking
6 Underestimates time needed to complete a task
7 Doesn't respond when spoken to
8 Has trouble getting started on a task
9 Has trouble dealing with frustration
10 Doesn't plan ahead

Discuss Aspects of Good Communication

Many different theories and constructs exist regarding what makes for "good" (i.e., effective) interpersonal communication, such that entire academic books are dedicated to the topic (e.g., Hargie, 2011). The scope of the literature is simply too broad to consider fully here, and certainly too extensive to discuss effectively with your client. However, one can distill several principles that seem to be consistently noted as important to being a good communicator (see Box 2). We recommend opening your conversation with the client here with a simple prompt (see Dialogue 2).

Dialogue 2

Therapist: *One thing is for sure, and that is that communication styles and behaviors have an effect on our relationships. People have lots of different ideas about what makes communication more or less effective, and I have some ideas in mind to talk about related to that. First, though, I'd like to ask … what do you think are the keys to effective communication?*

See what the client comes up with. Chances are that they will have some thoughts that map onto the kinds of aspects that are described in Box 2. Use these as springboards to a more thorough discussion about effective (and ineffective) elements of communication, making sure to at least incorporate some brief description of each one of the five qualities.

Box 2   Principles of Effective Communication Skills

Aspects of effective communication include:

- **Appropriateness.** There are unwritten social rules that govern when, what, and how we should communicate with others. Inappropriate interpersonal behavior or communication violates these rules, and tends to be received poorly. For instance, there is no written rule that changing the subject of conversation prematurely is forbidden, but if someone does this it tends to be frowned upon (unless there is an urgent reason behind it). Other similar behaviors include saying "hello" when one first sees someone, taking turns in conversation (and respecting that), and starting new topics of conversation when old ones seem finished.
- **Achieving a Goal.** Communication is generally goal- (or need-) driven. At a restaurant, customers communicate to get food. In a relationship, one partner may communicate to another to figure out what the couple will do the upcoming weekend. Communication that is confusing or unclear, or that has an emotional tone that is off-putting or incongruous with the situation, often fails to achieve its goal.
- **Strengthening a Relationship.** There are several types of communication behaviors that tend to strengthen relationships. One of them is being attentive and perceptive to both verbal and nonverbal messages, and then responding in a way that acknowledges these. This involves empathy, too, or understanding another's perspectives and feelings and then using that awareness to speak and behave in a congruent manner. Active listening behaviors are strongly related to this characteristic.
- **Expressiveness.** Similar to but more specific than goal achievement, effective communication conveys certain internal feelings or states, depending on the context. For instance, certain verbal and nonverbal behaviors communicate openness and willingness to converse, and to listen. We might broadly call this approachability. Related behaviors can include using direct eye contact, leaning forward in a conversation, having a smile, and nodding as a conversation partner speaks.
- **Assertiveness.** This should not be confused with aggression. Assertive communication appropriately communicates and advocates for ones needs and/or desires, and also encompasses a willingness to talk about difficult things, as well. Asking one's boss directly for a raise in a performance review meeting that has gone well is an example of appropriate assertiveness.

It is entirely possible in this exercise that you will discover that your client has a pretty good knowledge of the types of things that *are* appropriate to achieving good communication. Research on children with ADHD, in particular, shows that their *knowledge* of prosocial behavior is not that lacking, but instead it's their *implementation* of those behaviors that can be problematic. As such, your conversation may naturally turn to inquiring about the client's perceptions of how well they do actually communicate, and examples of times in their (recent or past) life they have noticed that they have *not* been a successful communicator. As this session mainly focuses on psychoeducation, it is not the moment to address any apparent weaknesses that the person expresses, but instead acknowledge the perceptiveness of the client, reinforce it, and make note of it as it may guide choice of future material. Use motivational interviewing techniques here to build the clients desire to improve communication in subsequent sessions.

Discuss Homework and Schedule Next Session

Suggested homework for clients after this session, to build awareness and (in many cases) prepare for subsequent sessions, include:

- Complete *Interpersonal Competence Questionnaire* (see Appendix B; Buhrmester et al., 1988)
- Complete *Conflict Resolution Styles Inventory* (see Appendix B; Kurdek, 1994)

References

Buhrmester, D., Furman, W., Wittenberg, M.T., & Reis, H.T. (1988). Five domains of interpersonal competence in peer relationships. *Journal of Personality and Social Psychology, 55*(6), 991–1008. 10.1037/0022-3514.55.6.991

Hargie, O. (Ed.). (2011). *Skilled Interpersonal Communication: Research, Theory and Practice* (5th ed.). Routledge/Taylor & Francis Group.

Kurdek, L.A. (1994). Conflict resolution styles in gay, lesbian, heterosexual nonparent, and heterosexual parent couples. *Journal of Marriage and Family, 56*, 705–722. 10.2307/352880

Robin, A.L., & Payson, E. (2002). The impact of ADHD on marriage. *The ADHD Report, 10*, 9–14. https://doi.org/abs101521adhd103920553

Session 2: Changing Behaviors to be Satisfied in my Personal Relationships

Corresponds to Module 5.1 of the *Thriving in College* Student Workbook

Session Outline

1 Check-in with client(s)
2 Set agenda
3 Review client's difficulties in personal relationships
4 Discuss skills of a good partner or friend
5 Practice indicated relationship behaviors (role plays)
6 Discuss homework
7 Schedule next session

Session Organization

Administration Format

Session 1 can be administered in a group or individual format. A group session may be optimal in that the presence of other students with ADHD may validate some of the shared experiences about relationships. However, the session can also be efficiently and effectively employed for an individual client, if a group format is not practical.

Materials Needed

The therapist should have a whiteboard, flipchart, or a projected digital document to capture group ideas and/or present material and a list of or handout with "take home messages" regarding the session's content, as well as instructions/goals for at-home work prior to the next session

- Copies of the Relational Worksheet (see later and Appendix A) are also needed.

As always, therapists are reminded to instruct clients ahead of the session to bring a notebook or device in which they can take notes. Also, it will be important for the client to have the completed *Interpersonal Competency*

DOI: 10.4324/9781003149590-24

Questionnaire and the *Conflict Resolution Styles Inventory* (Appendix B, completed in prior session) as this will help to inform your work in this session.

Session Content

Check-in with Client(s)

It is unlikely that this will be the first technique or content-heavy session that a client has done with you. Check-in time can be used to solicit brief discussion about homework or issues that the client is dealing with currently, or simply to see how things are going and strengthen rapport. In the event that this session is the first meeting with clients, check-in might focus more on feelings and expectations about therapy. In any event, aim for this to be brief (< 5 minutes), encouraging client(s) to postpone any additional discussion of this sort until after the session content is completed. See therapist-client check-in dialogue example in Skill 1: Session 1 as a model for this interaction, if needed. In the likely event that you have just completed Skill 5: Session 1, check in to make sure the client has completed and brought the inventories that were assigned as homework, as these will be used in this session. We also recommend having your client complete the *Progress Tracker* (see Appendix B), and briefly touching base on any declines or improvements in school functioning.

Set Agenda

Introduce the agenda for this session to the client (see Session Outline). It is helpful to have a visual aid to refer to, such as a flip chart or projected PowerPoint slide or printed handout. At this time, it might also be helpful to remind clients to write notes regarding important points in a therapy notebook. Setting the agenda should be speedily completed (< 2 minutes). See therapist-client agenda-setting dialogue example in Skill 1: Session 1 as a model, if needed.

Review Client Difficulties in Personal Relationships

A beginning point for this activity will be to review the interpersonal behaviors questionnaires that the clients completed as homework for Skill 5 Session 1 (see earlier). Use of negative conflict resolution styles (e.g., confrontative, overly assertive or critical, dismissing, or avoidant) will not be unusual, and the same goes for interpersonal competence difficulties (Canu et al., 2014). Moreover, research suggests that people with ADHD may be less aware of these behavioral patterns and their related fallout than others are (Owens et al., 2007). It is therefore important to anticipate that there may be some results from these questionnaires that are not particularly easy for the client to absorb, and this should be handled with sensitivity. Patterns that might be expected, given the existent literature on relational issues in colleges students and adults with

ADHD (e.g., Canu & Carlson, 2003; Canu et al., 2014; Sacchetti & Lefler, 2017; Wymbs & Molina, 2015; Wymbs et al., 2021) include:

- **Students with elevated inattentive (IA) symptoms** of ADHD may tend to score low on Initiation and Emotional Support scales on the *Interpersonal Competencies Questionnaire* (ICQ), and on the *Conflict Resolution Styles Inventory* (CRSI) may score low on the Positive Problem Solving scale and high on self-protection and acceptance.
- **Students with elevated hyperactivity-impulsivity (HI)** may also tend to score low on the Emotional Support ICQ scale, but also low on Conflict Management as well as high on Negative Assertion, Initiation, and Disclosure scales. They also may have low scores on the Positive Problem Solving CRSI scale, with high scores on Conflict Engagement, too.

These types of patterns are predictable given that those with the predominantly inattentive style of ADHD have been observed to have a somewhat passive and "tuned out" type of interpersonal style, whereas those whose ADHD includes high HI tend to act impulsively in social situations and also tend to express more emotional dysregulation, which comes with episodes of quick and intense anger or frustration that colors social interaction. Altogether, both main clusters of ADHD are often associated with more use of negative conflict and interpersonal behaviors and less use of positive ones.

Critical elements to reviewing the patterns of behavior that are noted by your client(s) will be to (a) affirm that nobody is perfect when it comes to interacting with others, or even those they are very close to, and (b) that *knowing* one's strengths *and* weaknesses is ultimately important to interpersonal growth and success. To these ends, engage your client in a discussion about how they perceive their interactive styles play out in both their friendships and their romantic relationships (see Dialogue 1). This will set the stage for discussion of positive relational skills (given later), and give the client a chance to reflect on things that they may personally want to change.

Dialogue 1

Therapist: So, let's talk about the work you did since last session, completing those questionnaires about interpersonal styles and conflict resolution patterns. What sorts of things stood out to you?

Client: Well, those were an eye-opener. Sheesh, I really never realized how bad I am at this.

Therapist: I see. Yeah, I think that lots of people have the same thought when they do these, whether they have ADHD or not. The truth is that these things can be hard for us to notice, until we sit down and actually do something like this.

Client:	*Really?*
Therapist:	*You bet! As we talk about this, I want you to remember that, truly, there is nobody who is "perfect" when it comes to interaction styles, nobody who doesn't sometimes use a not-so-great conflict resolution strategy. The important thing to gain from this is awareness. I mean, after all, how can anyone improve on anything if they don't know where to start?*
Client:	*Alright …* (takes a deep breath). *So one of the things that stood out is that I was low on the emotional support. That kind of stung. I kind of tend to think that it's best to stay out of family problems that someone else is having … actually, I think I kind of ignore them, or even say something like "well, that's on you" … but I see how that's really not very supportive, now. It's kind of like that with problems that I'm not really personally invested in that a friend is having, too … when these get brought up, I kind of zone out.*
Therapist:	*OK … that's good insight that you're having. I don't think you're the only one who does this, by the way … but can you see how this is something that might be annoying or even hurtful for someone else? What would it feel like for someone else to dismiss your problems?*
Client:	*The truth is that I talk about my problems with my parents all the time, and I get kind of hurt and frustrated when friends say things like "I'm sure it'll work out" or just change the subject. So, yeah, I can see how this could be a sticking point for someone else, too.*
Therapist:	*It can be easy sometimes to forget to take others' perspectives into account … for you, and for other people, too. I bet that they don't want to frustrate you, just like I bet you don't want to frustrate them.*
Client:	*Yeah … but I guess I'd like to be more emotionally supportive, anyway.*
Therapist:	*Good! We can work on strategies to change the way you interact with your friends and others, so they feel more emotionally supported. What else particularly stood out for you in those questionnaires?*
Client:	*OK, so, ha, not much that was good … I really identified with the questions that were about withdrawing from conflict resolution, but also with the negative conflict strategies.*
Therapist:	*So, you've mentioned that you are in a romantic relationship … I wonder whether you see these things playing out there?*
Client:	*Yeah, my partner is always saying that I pull a "hit-and-run" in our fights. I think it's pretty hard for them to deal with. We've come so close to breaking up so many times … I feel like I'm constantly begging for forgiveness. Yeah, I just suck at relationships.*
Therapist:	*I hear you being pretty upset now, too … like this is not something that you want to continue.*
Client:	*Exactly! It's happened before, too … I've been with good people over the years, and messed those relationships up … I don't want to do it again.*

Therapist:	*That is a good place to start ... we can work with that. Speaking of having things to work with, I wonder whether this process reminded you of any things that you do pretty well in your relationships?*
Client:	*Things I do well? Let's see ...* (looks through questionnaires) *well, the one questionnaire said that I was pretty engaging. I mean my initiation score was high. Maybe that's something that other people would like.*
Therapist:	*OK ... is that something that others have commented on, ever?*
Client:	*Actually, yes ... in fact, sometimes in those deep, late-at-night kinds of conversations that me and my friends or my partner and I have, the conversation turns to things like "why do you like me, anyway?" One of the first things that people say about me usually is that I'm fun, I'm always coming up with things to do.*
Therapist:	*I think this is a good example of how we all have strengths and weaknesses that we bring to our relationships. It's important not to lose sight of that, and to keep that aspect of yourself even as we work toward being more supportive of others.*

Discuss Skills of a Good Partner or Friend

There are, of course, lots of things that individuals do that affect the nature of their relationships, both in positive and negative ways. A lot of how people get along with one another is idiosyncratic to each dyad, or to the group. For instance, it's not totally uncommon for teenage friend groups to regularly refer to each other in derogatory terms, with a kind of mutual understanding that this is a signal of acceptance and membership, as opposed to rejection. Still, research has shown that there are particular types of behaviors that tend to be associated with satisfaction in and maintenance of friendships and romantic relationships, including the following.

1 **Positive conflict resolution.** This may be the single most important aspect of relational behavior when it comes to predicting relationships that last, and particularly so for marriages and other long-term romantic relationships (Gottman & Driver, 2005; Gottman & Levenson, 2000). In brief, *non-hostile engagement* with the partner (e.g., responsive conversation, non-verbal affirmations) and *productive focus on the conflict* (e.g., keeping topic focused on understanding the situation, each others' perspectives, potential solutions) are important. Equally important is avoiding *excessive or harsh criticism* and also *withdrawal from one's partner* (i.e., failure to address the conflict). All of these things may be inherently difficult for people with ADHD, given their dispositional tendencies toward impulsivity, inattention, and emotional dysregulation. Relatedly, it is very important to mention here that physical or emotional interpersonal violence (IPV), something that, as

noted earlier in this skill module, ADHD individuals may be at risk for, is an extreme conflict resolution behavior that is absolutely impermissible. In both friendships and romantic partnerships, having the skill of recognizing that you are at the "boiling point" and then being able to implement self-soothing or physical distancing (or both, as in "taking five" to separate for a few minutes and to return to the discussion once cooled down) before IPV occurs is paramount.

2 **Open (and yet tactful!) communication.** This is in some ways the opposite of the passive conflict resolution strategy, and also overlaps to a degree with the construct of positive conflict resolution. Open communication may be something that some college students with the predominantly inattentive presentation of ADHD may have particular difficulty with, given behavioral trends of passivity and withdrawal that have been noted. In any intimate relationship, whether it is with a good friend or a romantic partner, being able to articulate one's own perspectives and views, wants and needs, is really important to satisfaction and also to mutual understanding. What is equally important in this, though, is that the message also not come across like a bomb. In other words, when opinions differ, or when one is not happy with something going on in the relationship – whether it be a single behavior or longstanding patterns – how the message is delivered matters greatly. For example, if a student with ADHD is at dinner with their romantic partner and is dissatisfied with that person scrolling through their Instagram feed, saying something like "You are just the worst! I can't believe you are ignoring me and just looking at that stupid device!" is likely to be antagonizing and hurtful, whereas an alternative like "Are you doing something important now? I really like it when it's just us two and we can talk together, and I was hoping we could do that now" expresses the student's sentiments with appropriate assertiveness, and also invites the partner to engage while respecting their needs, too. Similarly, the use of *I-messages* provides an easy framework for phrasing potentially charged messages in order to accurately convey feelings but also frame it specifically and not put undo responsibility on the partner or friend. These messages (a) communicate the feeling the person has, (b) specify the trigger/situation, and (c) invite discussion on how to change or offer a related suggestion. For instance, in the aforementioned situation, an I-message would be something like "*I feel* frustrated now, *when you are on your iPhone* and we haven't seen each other all day. *Is it possible for us to put aside our devices* for half-an-hour when we get together?"

3 **Being a good listener.** Good listeners are those who pay attention to their conversation partners and to the content and flow of the conversation itself. This is often communicated by *observable behaviors*, some of which are automatic or nearly so (e.g., leaning slightly in toward a partner, naturally matching one's voice tone to that of the partner, certain non-verbal behavior like nodding at appropriate intervals) and others that are more voluntary

(e.g., asking an appropriate follow-up question, reflecting what a person has just said, offering an empathic response like "that seems like it's hard for you"). Again, these are things that people with ADHD inherently have difficulty with, given that inattention leads to mind wandering and/or off-task (i.e., off-conversation) behaviors, and that impulsivity can sometimes take the form of interrupting or changing subjects abruptly. Unfortunately, this can lead not only to hurt feelings or frustration on the part of a partner but also to low comprehension of the issue at stake on the part of the student with ADHD. When one is not skilled at this kind of engagement, trying to shift toward good listening may seem fairly artificial (e.g., "You mean I have to repeat back what someone says to me?"), a hurdle that you should be aware of in working with your client(s). It is thereby important to convey how employing these sorts of behaviors will help friends and partners to feel more understood, a key component of emotional support, and that active focus on these sorts of things does help one to better connect with and understand others, which can guide adaptive social behavior.

4 **Reciprocity.** There are multiple definitions of reciprocity. One way to think about this is specific to conversations. How does it feel to you when conversations seem entirely one-sided? When your partner or friend dictates all of the topics, or seems to just want to talk about themself? Again, here there is some overlap with another concept, that of being a good listener; it is impossible to be a good listener when one is doing all of the talking. Therefore, conscious *turn taking* in conversations is key (e.g., "So that sums up how my day went … how was yours?"). To take this further, it is usually appreciated when someone *actively solicits* the opinion or thoughts of a conversation partner (e.g., "Does that fit with your schedule tonight?"). Reciprocity can also be thought of as *giving back what you get* in a relationship. For instance, if a friend took several hours to help with a repair job on your car, it makes sense that when that friend communicates a need for help with some similarly onerous task that you would come to their aid. One easy way to think about reciprocity is to invoke the proverbial "Golden Rule" – do unto others as you would have them do unto you. In relationships, burdens are best shared, instead of being shouldered by only one partner (or friend). This is a skill that involves attention, perspective taking, and sometimes inhibition of automatic behavioral or cognitive responses (e.g., considering a matter settled when a friend nods as you describe plans for a weekend activity, rather than actively checking the person's opinion).

5 **Attention to others' wants and needs.** All of the four skills noted so far also have relevance when it comes to this point: If one does not *take care of one's friends and partners*, there is a good chance that they will begin to feel unappreciated, and to have less investment, satisfaction, and interest in continuing the relationship. Wants and needs can be both long-term and situational, and particularly the latter kind can be indicated by relatively

subtle behavioral cues and in fact contradict the former. For instance, one might be aware that one's partner is generally introverted, and that extended group activities (e.g., dinner parties) can be taxing. With this in mind, one may need to be sensitive to cues that the romantic partner is getting tired of being at a party, as well as other indicators that the person is really engaged and energized by a particular interaction and may want to stay longer. Other wants and needs may seem at first glance to be much more obvious. If a friend is sick, it is a nice and supportive thing to bring them a meal. If a partner has just been fired from a job, it is kind and potentially helpful to offer to talk about it, and to see what you can do to support them. There are lots of wants and needs that are more subtle: Needs to feel understood and appreciated, to feel loved, to pursue activities and life paths that are satisfying. What is really important to beginning to hone in on when these are salient is good perspective taking. Students might be coached to ask themselves, "how would I feel in this situation? What would I want or need?" While not a perfect barometer of someone else's internal desires, this thought exercise can be particularly helpful when the student senses some sort of disconnect or frustration on the part of their friend or partner, and to know what to do to work toward being supportive. The use of *if-then queries* can be really helpful in these cases (e.g., "If I were in your shoes, then I would probably want to just unwind. Instead of heading out right away to grocery shop, would you like me to make you some tea? We could talk about it some more, too, if you want."

Take some time to talk about each of these positive relational behaviors with your client. Describe what they are, and check in with them about how well they think they do these things. If the client is having difficulty in a particular kind of relationship or with a particular person, using that as a prompt for the client to think concretely about their behaviors may be very helpful. Drawing out examples of when they *did* and *did not* use some of these behaviors, and what the consequences were, can help the client to see the potential benefit of change, and can also help you to develop an idea of which behaviors you may want to focus on in the role-play practice (next) and in homework assignments for the future. We have included a Relational Worksheet in Appendix A that may help to facilitate this topic.

Practice Indicated Relationship Behaviors

At this juncture, your client has very likely indicated that they have not fully mastered implementing at least one of the five key relationship skills that are noted earlier. In-session role play can be useful to help demonstrate these skills and also to better specify deficiencies in a tailored fashion. In these role plays, which should be the focus for the remainder of the session, the most productive approach may be for you to use one of the situations that the client has already identified (i.e., a situation that really happened that the client nominates as problematic) as a model and training experience for *how to interact more effectively*. So, for instance, if the client has told you that in a recent interaction with their romantic partner, that person ended the conversation by saying "I just feel like you never listen to me" and then going into another room and closing the door, it may be clear that *being a good listener* and/or *paying attention to others' wants and needs* are skills that the client really needs to work on. An appropriate role play experience for this situation might unfold outlined in Dialogue 2.

Dialogue 2

Therapist: *So now what I think we should do is to practice some of these skills so that you can get the feel for them and then start to consciously use them more often in real life, so that things aren't so rocky in your relationships. Maybe we can use your recent interaction with Alonzo* [client's significant other] *as something to work with, first?*

Client: *Yeah, that might be good. That went pretty badly and I don't want to have that happen again.*

Therapist: *I hear you. It certainly sounded like it ended that night on a real down note. So, if I heard you right, it sounded like you two were sitting on the couch, you had just finished watching the movie, and then you were talking about what to do that weekend. Remind me of what happened next.*

Client: *Well, Alonzo started talking about some hike that a few of his friends had done recently. I kind of spaced out when he went on about it, I was kind of still thinking about the movie and feeling kind of hungry and wondering what we had to snack on. Then he said "does that sound good to you? I'm not sure what you are thinking." I had no idea what he'd really been talking about, and I just blurted out something like "I dunno, I kind of lost the thread, there, you were going on and on about your friends' hike and I am feeling hungry and I thought maybe we could make a snack and talk about the movie a bit?" Well, it turns out that Alonzo had been saying that he really missed connecting with these friends and wanted to invite them to do a new hike with us and how it was important to him that I and his friends should get to know each other and get along. He was trying to tell me what he needed ... and I just brushed it aside. He was so pissed. Yeah, I actually slept on the couch that night ... .*

Therapist: *Dang, yeah, I'm sorry, that sounds like it was hard.*

Client: *It really was. I didn't know if we were still going to be together the next day, honestly.*

Therapist: *So ... thinking about the relationship skills that we just discussed ... are there any that come to mind that you think you didn't use effectively in this interaction with Alonzo?*

Client: I think definitely not being a good listener. For sure. And also probably not paying attention to his needs. The fact is that we have been doing way more stuff with my friends than his ... and I never really tuned into that.

Therapist: OK, good. I think you're onto the right track. So, how do you think you could be a better listener with Alonzo, if you had to do this over?

Client: Well, first off, I would try to consciously orient myself more toward him and what he was saying. Like, for instance, I would have turned to face him more as he talked. And I would have watched him, and his expressions and stuff. I also think that if I said things like "yeah, that's a good idea" and "right, I want that too" and "sounds good to me" he would have known that I was really listening and also that I really wanted to be supportive, change things some, so that his need to stay connected with his other friends is taken care of.

Therapist: I think that this sounds like a really good plan. I know it's hard when you have ADHD to pay attention for a long period of time, but in conversations – unlike in class, a lot of the time – you can be using these active engagement strategies that really should keep your attention centered where you want it to be. That helps Alonzo to know you're still there with him, and also helps you to recognize his needs and to have a chance to respond supportively. So, you think you can do this ... and do you think it will help?

Client: Yeah ... I want to do those things. I know it will help.

Therapist: Awesome. OK, let's do this. Let's pretend that I am Alonzo, and you are back in this situation. I want you to use these skills, and see how it feels. OK?

Client: Alright, sure.

Therapist: Great, let's give this a try, see how it feels for you. I'll start. (Now as Alonzo) *That was a really great movie, I'm glad we chose that! You know, there's something that I've just been thinking about that I want to run by you. A few of the guys went and did this awesome hike the other day, they were telling me about. My buddy Nate said that it's called the Profile Trail. It sounded so cool ... .*

Client: Oh, wow ... so what did they say?

Therapist: (Aside to client) *That was good!* (Now as Alonzo again) *Well, it is over on Grandfather Mountain, and a pretty strenuous hike. There were some parts that even required ladders.*

Client: Ladders?! What for?

Therapist: (Aside to client) *Good!* (Now as Alonzo again) *Well, they said those areas were so rough and so steep that ladders were the only safe way to continue. Pretty cool, huh? So, after that ...* (Therapist completes description of trail, in long detail, reinforcing client's active listening as it occurs). *So, anyway, it all sounded really cool, like something maybe we would want to do sometime. But, honestly what it*

	really made me think about is how much I miss doing things with my buds. I mean, I really, really like you … and love the time we spend together … and I like your friends, too, we've done fun things with them. But I kind of feel like we never do things with my friends, and all this time away from them, I feel kind of disconnected. Is it OK with you if we do some things with them? I'd like you to get to know them, for us all to get along and stuff. I think it would help me reconnect with them. Maybe we could invite them to camp with us next weekend? Does that sound good to you?
Client:	*Yeah, babe … I'd like that. I don't mean to keep you away from your friends.*
Therapist:	(Still as Alonzo) *Oh, that's great! I think you're really going to like them! Hey, thanks a lot for listening. I really appreciate it.*
Client:	(Exhales hard.) *Oh, man, I'm kind of getting goosebumps just pretending here … it actually feels really good to even hear you pretend to be him and say "thanks for listening."*
Therapist:	*What does that do for you? What are you thinking and feeling, now?*
Client:	*I'm thinking that this is what being a good partner is like … and that I can do it! I'm kind of feeling like … somehow more connected … more caring … I dunno it just feels good in a hopeful kind of way. I think I've always been a lousy friend, and most of my relationships always seem to end badly, and maybe I've got it in me to change.*
Therapist:	*Yes, yes, I think you have it in you, too! Do you think you can actually now try to practice this next time you are with Alonzo? See how it feels in real life?*
Client:	*Yeah, I do. Let's do this!*

It is beyond the scope of this manual to provide you with detailed role play information for all the possible relational skills and situations that clients may bring to the session, but hopefully this example adequately illustrates the type of interaction you may have. It will be up to you to tailor this successfully to the specific needs of your clients(s). Depending on their comfort with the skills that you are trying to impart in this role play, you may need to invent new scenarios to provide additional role play practice. Again, depending on the needs of your client, you may take the role of their friend or partner, or, and particularly for clients whose skill level is quite deficient, play the role *of the client*, modeling adaptive skills as the client role plays their partner.

Discuss Homework and Schedule Next Session

As suggested at the end of the role play mentioned earlier, the main practice exercises that the client will do after this session are putting the relational skills to use in their real life. The most effective way for them to do this is to use a kind of journal to track (a) the skills that they intentionally were trying and also (b) how they perceive those to have worked in specific relational situations. This often accentuates positive social reinforcement (e.g., partner spontaneously saying they feel heard), and also provides grist for follow-up in future sessions for fine-tuning and or troubleshooting. A basic worksheet that can be used is included in Appendix A.

References

Canu, W.H., & Carlson, C.L. (2003). Differences in heterosocial behavior and outcomes of ADHD-symptomatic subtypes in a college sample. *Journal of Attention Disorders, 6*(3), 123–133. 10.1177/108705470300600304

Canu, W.H., Tabor, L.S., Michael, K.D., Bazzini, D.G., & Elmore, A.L. (2014). Young adult romantic couples' conflict resolution and satisfaction varies with partner's attention-deficit/hyperactivity disorder type. *Journal of Marital and Family Therapy, 40*(4), 509–524. 10.1111/jmft.12018

Gottman, J.M., & Driver, J.L. (2005). Dysfunctional marital conflict and everyday marital interaction. *Journal of Divorce & Remarriage, 43*(3–4), 63–78. 10.1300/J087v43n03_04

Gottman, J.M., & Levenson, R.W. (2000). The timing of divorce: Predicting when a couple will divorce over a 14-year period. *Journal of Marriage and the Family, 62*(3), 737–745. 10.1111/j.1741-3737.2000.00737.x

Owens, J.S., Goldfine, M.E., Evangelista, N.M., Hoza, B., & Kaiser, N.M. (2007). A critical review of self-perceptions and the positive illusory bias in children with ADHD. *Clinical Child and Family Psychology Review Volume 10*, pp. 335–351.

Sacchetti, G.M., & Lefler, E.K. (2017). ADHD symptomology and social functioning in college students. *Journal of Attention Disorders, 21*(12), 1009–1019. 10.1177/1087054714557355

Wymbs, B.T., & Molina, B.S.G. (2015). Integrative couples group treatment for emerging adults with ADHD symptoms. *Cognitive and Behavioral Practice, 22*(2), 161–171. 10.1016/j.cbpra.2014.06.008

Wymbs, B.T., Canu, W.H., Sacchetti, G.M., & Ranson, L.M.(2021). Adult ADHD and Romantic Relationships: What we know and what we can do to help. *Journal of Marital and Family Therapy, 47*(3), 664–681. 10.1111/jmft.12475

Session 3: (Re)negotiating a Positive Relationship with Parents

Corresponds to Module 5.2 of the *Thriving in College* Student Workbook

Session Outline

1 Check-in with client(s)
2 Set agenda
3 Discuss how parents interacted with the client in childhood and adolescence
4 Discuss how this relationship has changed and any difficulties that have emerged
5 Discuss ways in which parents can still be helpful and what the client wants
6 Discuss how to talk with parents about changing relationship
7 Discuss homework
8 Schedule next session

Session Organization

Administration Format

Session 3 can be administered in a group or individual format. A group session may be optimal in that the presence of other students with ADHD may validate some of the shared experiences and difficulties that individual clients may have in their relationships with parents. However, the session can also be efficiently and effectively employed for an individual client, if a group format is not practical.

Materials Needed

The therapist should have a whiteboard, flipchart, or a projected digital document to capture group ideas and/or present material and a list of or handout with "take home messages" regarding the session's content, as well as instructions/goals for at-home work prior to the next session might be desirable.

- Copies of the *Parental Authority Questionnaire* are also needed (see later and Appendix B).

DOI: 10.4324/9781003149590-25

As always, therapists are reminded to instruct clients ahead of the session to bring a notebook or device in which they can take notes.

Session Content

Check-in with Client(s)

It is unlikely that this will be the first technique or content-heavy session that a client has done with you. Check-in time can be used to solicit brief discussion about homework or issues that the client is dealing with currently, or simply to see how things are going and strengthen rapport. In the event that this session is the first meeting with clients, check-in might focus more on feelings and expectations about therapy. In any event, aim for this to be brief (< 5 minutes), encouraging client(s) to postpone any additional discussion of this sort until after the session content is completed. See therapist-client check-in dialogue example in Skill 1: Session 1 as a model for this interaction, if needed. We also recommend having your client complete the *Progress Tracker* (see Appendix B), and briefly touching base on any declines or improvements in school functioning.

Set Agenda

Introduce the agenda for this session to the client (see earlier). It is helpful to have a visual aid to refer to, such as a flip chart or projected PowerPoint slide or printed handout. At this time it might also be helpful to remind clients to write notes regarding important points in a therapy notebook. Setting the agenda should be speedily completed (< 2 minutes). See therapist-client agenda-setting dialogue example in Skill 1: Session 1 as a model, if needed.

Discuss How Parents Interacted with the Client in Childhood and Adolescence

As has been reviewed before (see introduction to Skill 5 and Session 1), relationships between parents and their children with ADHD can be strained – more so and more often than in families without ADHD. Parents of children with diagnosed ADHD often have to tag on the burden of (a) navigating in-school accommodations and added communication with teachers and staff, (b) medical treatment of ADHD, often involving extensive titration and reformulation of medications, (c) implementing behavioral interventions at home to facilitate more positive and adaptive behavior, and (d) simply maintaining a positive and helpful stance with a child (or children) who has the core characteristics of inattention, hyperactivity-impulsivity, and emotional dysregulation.

One parenting style that emerges in those with ADHD children with more frequency is *permissive*, which tends to simply let disruptive behavior continue without correction. This, of course, is not optimal for the development of generally adaptive behavior. Another style that more often emerges in the presence of ADHD is *authoritarian*, which tends toward punitive, overly-critical, and non-cooperative behavior on the part of parents. Evidence suggests that such types of parenting may exacerbate ADHD symptoms as well as comorbid disruptive behavior, as seen in Oppositional Defiant Disorder and/or Conduct Disorder (ODD/CD; e.g., Johnston, 1996; Lindahl, 1998). Further, retrospective research of college students who report on the typical behaviors of their parents in childhood suggest, again, that maternal parenting styles in this specific subsection of the emerging adult ADHD population tended to be more authoritarian, and that this was associated with higher reported anxiety, depression, stress, and greater ADHD symptoms, as well (Stevens et al., 2019).

Optimally, as is the goal in many parent training interventions for ADHD, parents employ an *authoritative* style, which follows the tenets of setting logical and reasonable limits for child behavior, positively reinforcing adaptive behaviors, and collaboratively understanding and approaching disruptive behavior for change. Parents that raise children and adolescents with ADHD in this way tend to assist their children by providing adaptive "scaffolding." In developmental psychology, the concept of scaffolding involves giving children as much support as they need, but not more than they need, and then gradually reducing the support so that the child can develop their own skills. This concept has relevance for adolescents and emerging adults with ADHD in that parents often have difficulty figuring out just how much support to provide. For example, helping to organize their schoolwork and other daily tasks (e.g., by setting expectations about where and when homework is done) may facilitate short-term success, but could also hamper the personal development of coping skills if this help is provided for longer than needed. Thus, an optimal amount of scaffolding (i.e., just enough support and not too much) can be considered characteristic of an authoritative parenting style. One of the things that we recommend to help facilitate a discussion with your client(s) about their childhood and adolescent experiences with their parents is to complete the Parental Authority Questionnaire (Buri, 1991), which is included in Appendix B. This 30-item inventory is quickly completed and scored, and provides the client with a perspective on what type(s) of parenting they experienced in childhood, which you can then reflect on and discuss (see Dialogue 1).

Dialogue 1

Therapist: Thanks for taking the time to complete this questionnaire … I was wondering what you found out when you scored it?

Client: Well, kind of a mix of things … basically, it said that my mom used mostly an authoritative parenting style, and my dad was more permissive than anything else.

Therapist: Are those results consistent with your own memory about childhood and teen years at home?

Client: Pretty much, although I would say it kind of fluctuated for my dad over time. I remember situations from early in my childhood where I would say he really was into "tough love," kind of more authoritarian than anything else. I think after a while when that approach – which, to be fair, I think he grew up with – didn't work, he just kind of threw up his hands and gave up trying with me. I mean, he still loved me … I don't think he doesn't … just became a lot more hands-off.

Therapist: OK, well, it sounds like then, for you, that your mom was really the one who dealt with you and in other ways helped you as you grew up, until you left home. Is that right?

Client: Yeah, yeah I think so.

Therapist: OK, so the first step I think in reformulating your current relationship with your parents is to think about what both tended to do when you were at home, and then identify things that were helpful and others that were not. So … let's start with your dad … what things did he do, as a parent, that you found to be helpful to you in some way? What about other things that you thought were not helpful?

Client: Let's see … I think sometimes it was helpful that he would pretty much let me do what I wanted to do. It kind of helped me to learn to be independent, and to rely on myself, at least a little. The downside of that was that I didn't feel very connected to him. I also didn't really trust him … it's like he didn't exercise a lot of judgment. There were some things that he knew I was doing that he probably knew were a bad idea, but he didn't try to convince me to give up those things, and that ended up hurting me in some ways.

Therapist: That's fair. I'm glad that at least you can see some positive side to how he tended to interact with you. Alright, now let's consider your mom: What are things that she did that were helpful to you, and what about things that were not so helpful?

Client: Honestly, my mom did a lot for me that I know could not have been easy or fun for her but it got me through high school. Even after working all day, she would come home and then sit with me at my desk and talk through with me what homework I really needed to do that night, and help me plan how I would do it. She'd then check in on me, help to keep me accountable … sometimes even when

> *I would get mad and say she was overcontrolling. She would also do nice things for me when I made my goals ... like a lot of times she would bring me something to drink, like some cocoa, when I had finished one thing and had one to go. She'd also help me plan out bigger things that I got to do if I made bigger goals, like passing classes each quarter. She also wasn't super rigid about all of this ... if something cool or important came up and I really needed to skip a night of work or whatever, she would listen and usually be OK with that, or help me to think about which thing was actually more important, getting my work done or doing something with my friends, for instance.*
>
> Therapist: *Wow, sounds like she really helped you. In any of this were there things that she did that you felt were more harmful than helpful?*
>
> Client: *Well ... since I've been at college, it's been hard to stay on track sometimes. I think maybe that's because she did such a good job of helping me ... like I didn't really understand how much her being there made me successful in school.*

Discuss How the Relationship Has Changed and Any Difficulties that Have Emerged

Another key component in negotiating a new relationship with parents is to identify where the conflict points might be now, after the transition away to college. This is a big issue even for college students who are living at home while attending college – in fact, it might be even more salient in this situation. Both the parents and the young adult child (i.e., the college student) have to adjust to this new situation. The student obviously is likely to be dealing with a host of new tasks and responsibilities that parents at least facilitated if not outright took care of until they moved out of the home (or psychologically "graduated" to adult status in that same home). Parents have to acknowledge the newly earned independence of their adult child, and become comfortable having less oversight and giving less assistance. Both may also miss each other's company, quite a bit. Homesickness on the part of college students is quite common, and part of that may include a yearning for the care and help their parents traditionally gave them.

There's lots of opportunities for conflict in this situation. Parents who are used to knowing virtually everything their child does may seem overbearing, or intrusive. On the opposite side, children who are wanting to "live their life" may be seen as ungrateful, or deceptive, or aloof. Some parents could also feel that their child's requests for assistance are overly needy, and may contend that the college student should take more responsibility, including having a job to help with rent or tuition or other expenses (of course, this is a simple necessity for many). No matter what the pre-college history is, between parents and children, there is almost always a potential for strain in the relationship when college begins. Take a few minutes to talk through how this might be the case for your client. An opener like "So, since you've been in college, things have obviously changed a lot for you, perhaps including in your relationship with your parents. Have there been any things about this relationship that have bothered you?" is a good place to start. Common sources of strain in the relationship include:

- **Intrusiveness.** Students perceive that parents are wanting to know *too much* about their day-to-day lives at college.
- **Overprotection.** Students perceive that parents are trying to solve their problems, or are getting involved at the college or in their lives in unwanted ways.
- **Lack of communication.** Well-meaning parents may feel anxious about the adjustment of their child in college, and perceive the quantity/frequency of calls, texts, or other communication is lacking. This also may be construed by parents as a lack of caring.
- **Finances.** There may be disagreement between parents and their adult children as to who should pay for what.
- **Disconnection.** Parents and their children may feel like they lack common ground for meaningful conversations without the daily contact they are used to.

One thing to note: If your client says that there is really nothing that they perceive as being astray in their relationship with their parents … that's OK! While you might want to employ a gentle follow-up (e.g., "Really? No tension between you at all?"), remember that it may actually be the case that the student and their parent(s) are doing well together. It's OK to progress onto the next section … identifying how parents continue to be helpful to them … because actual formalization of expectations and boundaries is still important for the long-term health of this critical relationship.

Discuss Ways in Which Parents Can Still Be Helpful and What the Client Wants

There will likely be areas of strain in the relationship, and it is important as the therapist to acknowledge those your client reports. However, it's also important to refocus the conversation on what is still working, because it will likely become a central aspect of what the student wants in their relationship with their parents, going forward. Identifying these things, and then explicitly noting the things that the client would like to change, as well, are the heart of this step. It is strongly encouraged that you have your client take notes while this discussion goes on, and you may want to, as well, to help facilitate some final conclusions (see Dialogue 2). Your client should use paper and pen or laptop to note specific answers to and other thoughts related to the therapist's questions, which will be used later.

Dialogue 2

Therapist: *While it's clear that there are some things that are causing strife between you and your parents, it may be the case that this is not all of the picture, and we need to see that whole picture in order to successfully outline what you'd like from your relationship going forward. So, with that in mind, can you tell me about things that your parents are currently doing that you **do** find to be helpful, and that you might like them to continue?*

Client: *Sure. You're right, it's definitely not all bad. I would say that even though my mom annoys me when she checks up on every assignment or test that I mention, I don't mind her texts or calls. I can feel that she still loves me. That's nice ... I don't have a really big connection to others here at school, at least yet, and so that positivity really does feel good. I also appreciate that she and Dad do ask if I need anything, if I need money and stuff. Right now I'm good ... but it actually makes me stress less to know that they seem ready to be there for me if I need it.*

Therapist: *So it sounds like you really value the connection and supportiveness of your parents, but not the nagging.*

Client: *Yes.*

Therapist: *Is it safe to assume that's an aspect of your relationship that you wouldn't like to change?*

Client: *Yes. I mean, the amount of support with money and other material things that they give may be something ... well, I hope it will be something ... that can decrease over time. But the check-ins and stuff like that, yeah, I would like that to continue.*

Therapist: *OK, so what do these things look like, exactly? I mean, let's get down to what you actually want your interactions and their behaviors to look like. How many times a week do you think is right to be talking? Texting? And when is it OK to ask about things you're doing in class, and how? Is there a right and wrong way to ask, in your opinion?*

Client: *Huh, OK ... yeah, maybe it does help to think about this specifically. Alright, let's work on this ... .* (Client uses paper and pen or laptop to note specific answers to and other thoughts related to the therapist's questions, which will be used later.)

Discuss Maintaining Positive Feelings and Confidence in the Relationship

As noted earlier, from both the student and parent perspective, a lot is changing in the mutual relationship during the college years, and perhaps especially during the transition to college. The internal preference and drive for independence that emerging adults experience tends to be strong. With these as a contextual factor, parental "checking in" behaviors, which in many cases can be thought of as psychological replacements for simply being able to literally see what is going on with their child, can elicit strong emotional responses that might lead to confrontations or other negative communication. Another understandable reaction from the student may be to further distance themself from their parents, calling less often, not responding to texts, and otherwise checking out. This may lead to students only communicating with parents *when they need something* (e.g., more money on their meal plan card, need help resolving a problem with a roommate or professor), which can come off to parents as if all they are to their child is a walking wallet or support provider, or that their child is in real trouble and needs immediate assistance. Students often also do not share the *good* things that are happening, which can add to the latter impression. These patterns of communication, of course, are rather different from the partnership one strives for in a developing, friendly, adult relationship.

Of course, the problem with all of this is that it can put a real strain on the relationship, where the predominant experience is perceived as negative, potentially on both sides. Parents may begin to lose confidence that their child is being honest and forthright in their interactions. College students may begin to think that their parents lack trust in their ability to self-navigate, to deal with the challenges and make decisions that are necessary for success and happiness. Neither of these outcomes need to cast a permanent pall on things, but on the other hand it seems best, for everyone's well being, to avoid them.

So what are some of the things that you can coach your client to do, to help maintain positive feelings and confidence in their relationship with their parents? Well, fortunately, the same skills that are useful in being a good partner or friend, which were covered in the previous session, are applicable here. In fact, it might be that you want to quickly review those now. You could then ask your client to contemplate which of those skills (e.g., reciprocity) they think is important to employ in their relationship with their parents. Further, it is likely that helping the student to appreciate the perspective of their parents (e.g., still wanting to help, also probably feeling substantial sadness at their child departing) will also help the client to develop empathy, understanding, and maybe even patience for their parents' "annoying" behaviors. Encouraging your client to share both their successes and their difficulties might also go a way toward reassuring parents and developing a more balanced relationship. Additionally, this perspective can be very important in the actual negotiation of the new relationship. Requests for change can seem more like "demands" if there isn't any acknowledgment of the others' point of view. Finally, while college students are testing their proverbial wings and in many ways acting independently, it is still somewhat likely that support is still needed from parents, in some form, or at least that support may be needed further in the future. Maintaining a relationship marked more by happiness and closeness is much more likely to yield any needed support than one that is contentious or hostile. An example conversation on this topic is shown in Dialogue 3.

Dialogue 3

Therapist:	*So, one of the things that I've been hearing from you is annoyance about what you perceive as your parents' attempts to control your life. Am I right that at times you have felt mad about this?*
Client:	*For sure.*
Therapist:	*And do you think that made communication with your parents difficult?*
Client:	*Yes. I sometimes get angry, and tell them to stop, and then they get angry, and say that they don't know what to do with me anymore, and it kind of ends with nobody feeling great.*
Therapist:	*Hmm. Yeah, that doesn't sound fun, at all.*
Client:	*It's not!*
Therapist:	*So that's kind of why this renegotiation is important. Having mutual understandings about what is good for both sides and why they want it can help smooth things out between you.*
Client:	*I'd like that for sure. I also don't want to just give in and let them run my life like when I was in high school.*
Therapist:	*Right, I understand that. And maybe they don't want to do that either. I mean, let's think about their perspective a little. How long were they your parents before you left home for school?*
Client:	(Laughs.) *Well, Dr. Canu, it was about eighteen years!*
Therapist:	*So that's a long time. Is it fair to say that they are used to, for lack of a better way to put it, taking care of things for you?*
Client:	*Well, that's kind of fair. I mean, I did do some stuff for myself, more and more, as I got older. But yeah, I guess they have always taken care of at least some things for me.*
Therapist:	*So let's say that you had a job for 18 years, and then that job just kind of ended. Or, rather, it changed a lot. Do you think it would be easy to just stop doing things that you had done all that time?*
Client:	*I guess that's a fair point. It would take me a while, I bet.*
Therapist:	*Then there's another thing that may be harder for you to appreciate, just given your place in life. But maybe the example of a really good friend would work here, because this may have really happened … is there a time in your life where you were really close with someone, and then they moved away?*
Client:	*Sure. Yeah, it was actually when I came to college. My best friend, Jorge, went to a different university, in a different state, actually.*

Therapist:	*Was Jorge someone that you spent a lot of time with, before you both went to your different colleges?*
Client:	*Oh, totally. We saw each other literally every day. He was over at my house a lot, dinners, weekends, I was over at his house the same way, saw each other in school, we both ran cross country and track together, played Dungeons and Dragons in the same group together … yeah.*
Therapist:	*So, what was it like for you when you suddenly couldn't see him or spend time together?*
Client:	*I thought it would be a lot easier than it was, actually. It really sucked. I really missed him, just being able to talk about random things and laugh and know that I had someone who I liked … basically loved … and that I could be totally comfortable with.*
Therapist:	*Mmm hmm. Yeah, I'm sure that was tough. Really tough. How long had you known Jorge?*
Client:	*Since 2nd grade.*
Therapist:	*So 10 or 11 years? That's a long time.*
Client:	*Yeah.* (Sits with this.) *I miss him.*
Therapist:	*And you didn't even know him for 18 years.*
Client:	*Huh?* (Thinks.) *Oh. Wait. Right.* (Pauses.) *So you are trying to say that my parents may really, really miss me?*
Therapist:	*Yes. What do you think? Could that be behind why they act the way they do, sometimes?*
Client:	*I suppose so. The way I feel about Jorge, how it hurts not to be with my friend … I guess it could be way worse for them. Without me being there, I mean.*
Therapist:	*Uh huh. Do you think knowing that should make a difference in how you deal with them?*
Client:	*Maybe I should be more patient. Maybe I should cut them some slack, maybe meet them halfway and just be a little nicer.*

Discuss how to talk with Parents about Changing the Relationship

At this point, you and the client should have a better understanding of the history of their relationship with their parents, as well as things that are going right, and things that are not … which is all needed to formulate the "ask" for how the relationship can change to be more positive all around. We recommend getting pretty concrete here, and a good way to do this is simply to have the client use the following worksheet (Box 1) to document (a) how they want the relationship to change, (b) how they think their parents will think about it, and (c) things they should keep in mind about how to communicate about it. The worksheet essentially guides the student through this, point-by-point, which should also help structure the conversation with their parents.

Box 1   Changing my Relationship with my Parents

Thing I want to Change	How my Parents will Think About it	What I should keep in Mind While Asking
1.		
2.		
3.		
4.		
5.		

Coach your client to list these "asks" in rank-order, or, in other words, to put the thing they feel to be most important in #1, second most important in #2, and so on. Note that it is possible that your client can think of more than five things that they want to change about their relationship with their parents. We recommend, in such cases, having the client rank the top 3 to 5, and make a note of the others elsewhere, to hold for a later time. It is best if the conversation with their parents is focused and to the point, and not overwhelming. Identifying and working on several points for change will be plenty, in all likelihood, for a while, and meaningful change in those areas is likely to be experienced by the client as quite positive. Note that it is also possible that a client may only have 1 or 2 things they can identify that they really would like to change. That is fine! Work with the client to achieve the change they want.

With this worksheet in hand, your client will have what they want to ask for, but could still most likely use some coaching on how to do the asking. In addition to reminding the client about good relationship skills that they can employ that were addressed in the previous session (e.g., open communication, paying attention to wants and needs of others), here are some tips that you can pass along to give the conversation with their parents the best chance it can have of achieving positive change.

1 **Stress your desire to create and strengthen a sustainable relationship.** Students can convey to parents that they do not wish their relationship to be a contentious one. They can also convey that their needs and desires are different now that they are entering adulthood and living (in many cases) independently. This is something that almost necessitates change.

2 **Express thanks for what parents have done for you.** Hopefully, the perspective-taking exercises you have done will have suggested that in working for and living with and loving you over your entire life up to college has, whether they show it openly or not, made your parents feel exceedingly close to you. It has also been a lot of work. Express gratitude for these things!

3 **Realize that some of what they want is a maintained sense of closeness. How are you most comfortable doing that, while still being independent?** Now, you have moved away … and that can be experienced by them as moving on, a loss, and being left behind. Some of their "nosiness" may be a kind of reaching out, trying to maintain the relationship. Building in some ways to maintain connection with your parents may be a really good thing.

4 **Tell them that you are going to be OK … and also tell them that if you really need them, you will let them know.** Asking for independence, for less frequent calls, or more autonomy in your choices, is natural for a college student. This is easier to do for parents if they know that you will ask for help if you are in trouble. The help doesn't have to be "saving" you; it can be advice, or just listening and being supportive.

5 **Schedule a time with your parents to do this.** It shows them that you are serious, and that this is important. It would be nice if you could have this talk face-to-face … it's easier to see their reactions and know how it's being received. However, over the phone or by Zoom or Facetime would be fine. We do recommend not texting about this. Intent and feeling are things that are not always well understood in text communications.

6 Let your parents tell you their views and feelings, too. In other words, be a good listener!

7 Try to be concrete in negotiating what you want. In other words, if you want something different from your parents, try to communicate *what that actually looks like*. What behaviors can they engage in – or stop – in order for you and them both to know that they are meeting your needs as their adult child.

Discuss Homework and Schedule the Next Session

The main assignment coming out of this session is an actual discussion between the client and their parents about their relationship. It is suggested that the therapist gauge the comfort level of the client re: having the discussion, and bolster faltering or weak motivation by reminding the client of how proactively addressing this important life change will actually benefit both them and their parents in terms of satisfaction and mutual understanding. A mid-week (or post-session) check-in may be a good thing to schedule or establish, either through phone or electronic means. As needed, follow-up sessions on this topic may be employed; otherwise, scheduling additional sessions is contingent on other identified needs for the client (e.g., continuing to address professional/work relationship issues).

References

Buri, J.R. (1991). Parental authority questionnaire. *Journal of Personality Assessment, 57*(1), 110–119. 10.1207/s15327752jpa5701_13

Johnston C. (1996). Parent characteristics and parent-child interactions in families of non-problem children and ADHD children with higher and lower levels of oppositional-defiant behavior. *Journal of Abnormal Child Psychology, 24*(1), 85–104. 10.1007/BF01448375

Lindahl, K.M. (1998). Family process variables and children's disruptive behavior problems. *Journal of Family Psychology, 12*(3), 420–436. 10.1037/0893-3200.12.3.420

Stevens, A.E., Canu, W.H., Lefler, E.K., & Hartung, C.M. (2019). Maternal parenting style and internalizing and ADHD symptoms in college students. *Journal of Child and Family Studies, 28*(1), 260–272. 10.1007/s10826-018-1264-4

Skill 6: Managing Tasks of Daily Living or "Adulting"

(~3 sessions)

Corresponds to Skillset 6 of the *Thriving in College* Student Workbook

Background for the Therapist

In this manual, we have already addressed the connection between ADHD and difficulties in a number of areas of functioning (e.g., academics, personal relationships, physical health behaviors) for college students. In this final module, we will discuss the association between ADHD and difficulties in tasks of daily living. We begin with a brief overview of the existing research in this area, followed by discussion prompts for the therapist to assess problematic areas of daily living for the client. Finally, we offer a number of strategies to share with clients to help them manage and improve their tasks of daily living.

Tasks of daily living vary in immediate importance but are all necessary for satisfactory adaptation in adult life. If we consider the lives of most college students, there are lots of daily living tasks that they have to keep track of, including keeping a clean living space and doing laundry, organizing a home workspace or office, grocery shopping and food preparation, managing finances, errands and appointments, such as renewing a driver's license or making an appointment with the doctor, making travel/social plans, and, for some students, obtaining and keeping paid employment. It will come as no surprise that students with ADHD often have substantial difficulties in many of these areas due to deficits in executive functioning and problems with organization, time management, and planning. Emerging adults sometimes refer to these tasks or issues as "adulting."

The strategies for managing tasks of daily living that are shared in this module use and build on many of the skills previously addressed in this treatment program. We begin with an overview of research on the association of ADHD with impairment in tasks of daily living. Session 1 focuses on identifying specific non-career areas of "adulting" the client would like to work on, while Session 2 is designed to help the client identify and implement new (or old) skills and strategies to improving their functioning in key areas. Finally, Session 3 focuses specifically on job skills and career directions, given the importance of this area of functioning for most adults.

DOI: 10.4324/9781003149590-26

Student Workbook

If you are using the *Thriving in College* student workbook, you will find that Skillset 6 on *Adulting* corresponds to the material in this section. In this therapist guide, we recommend that you provide psychoeducation and then assess your client's specific needs for health and lifestyle skills in Session 1 and then tailor the content you emphasize accordingly. Together, Sessions 2 and 3 in this manual correspond to multiple modules in the workbook, allowing you to tailor skills information and skills practice opportunities to each client.

Therapist Guide Session	Workbook Modules
1	6.0 Why it Matters, Pre-Assessment, and Roadmap
2	6.1 Organizing Your Living Space and Keeping it Neat
	6.2 Planning Your Meals, Social Activities, and Appointments
	6.3 Managing Finances
3	6.4 Succeeding at Work and Career Prep

Session 1: How ADHD is Related to Impairment in Daily Life Activities and Identifying Areas for Improvement

Corresponds to Module 6.0 of the *Thriving in College* Student Workbook

Session Outline

1 Check-in with client(s)
2 Set agenda
3 Discuss ADHD and impairment in daily life activities
4 Facilitate client focus on own daily life adjustment
5 Discuss homework
6 Schedule next session

Session Organization

Administration Format

Session 1 should be administered in an individual format since the identification of what areas to focus on will be specific to each individual. Note that, first, this session will briefly review the types of daily life activities that college students with ADHD often struggle with and the ways that tasks of daily living might be impacted by ADHD. Second, there are a series of discussion prompts that will help you and your client identify which areas to work on during subsequent sessions of this module. As such, familiarity with the daily challenges associated with ADHD and also the direction of future sessions will help make for an effective session. Make sure to read this entire session's content, and if needed read further in an authoritative text regarding the nature of ADHD (e.g., Barkley's *Attention-Deficit/Hyperactivity Disorder: A Handbook for Diagnosis and Treatment*).

Materials Needed

Attending students should have a notebook or pad of paper to take notes. It may be helpful for the therapist to have some organizing visual materials, either in a projected PowerPoint, flipchart, or handouts.

DOI: 10.4324/9781003149590-27

Session Content

Check-in with Client

It is unlikely that this will be the first technique or content-heavy session that a client has done with you. Check-in time can be used to solicit brief discussion, or simply to see how things are going and build rapport. In the event that this session is the first meeting with clients, check-in might focus more on feelings and expectations about therapy. In any event, aim for this to be brief (< 5 minutes), encouraging for any additional discussion of this sort to be postponed until after the session content is completed. See therapist-client check-in dialogue example in Skill 1: Session 1 as a model for this interaction, if needed. We also recommend having your client complete the *Progress Tracker* (see Appendix B), and briefly touching base on any declines or improvements in school functioning.

Set Agenda

Introduce the agenda for this session to the client (see above). Again, it may be helpful to have a visual aid to refer to, such as a flip chart or projected PowerPoint slide or printed handout. At this time, it also might also be helpful to remind clients to write notes regarding important points in a therapy notebook. Setting the agenda should be speedily completed (< 2 minutes). See therapist-client agenda-setting dialogue example in Skill 1: Session 1 as a model, if needed.

Discuss ADHD and Impairment in Daily Life Activities

Given difficulties in other areas of functioning, it should come as no surprise that college students with ADHD often struggle with activities of daily living. These "adulting" activities include keeping a clean living space, doing laundry, organizing a home workspace, grocery shopping and food preparation, managing finances, making travel/social plans, and keeping up with errands and appointments, such as doctors' appointments to renew medication prescriptions. Some students may also wish to obtain a part-time job.

Successful completion of these activities requires organization, attention, planning, and other executive functioning skills that students with ADHD often struggle with, as we have discussed in prior modules. For example, the living and work space of a college student with ADHD might be extremely disorganized, leading to frequently misplacing items like keys, cell phone, wallet, bills, homework, and appointment reminders. Rather than planning ahead and grocery shopping for a weeks' worth of meals, an individual with ADHD might stop by the store daily, or worse, skip meals or frequently stop for fast food. A student with ADHD might have to dig through a pile of dirty laundry to find an outfit clean enough to wear to class. Existing research documents that individuals with ADHD have difficulties in many of these activities of daily living. For example, research shows that adults with ADHD have difficulty with time management, finances, and doing chores, compared to individuals without ADHD (Holst & Thorell, 2020).

Finally, research demonstrates difficulties related to employment for individuals with ADHD. For example, adults with ADHD report often not meeting their own work standards or achieving their potential at work (Fuermaier et al., 2021). Having ADHD is also associated with shorter duration of employment, being fired from a job, and changing jobs at a higher rate (Barkley, 2002). Further, employers often report lower work performance ratings for individuals with ADHD as compared to those without the disorder (Barkley, 2002).

Problems in these areas of daily living can exacerbate, and be exacerbated by, other difficulties that are common to college students with ADHD that we have already discussed in this manual. For example, not successfully managing grocery shopping can result in unhealthy eating behaviors, thus exacerbating poor physical health. Forgetting to fill or pick up a prescription for ADHD medications can result in unmanaged ADHD symptoms. Misplacing homework or materials needed for classes can perpetuate academic difficulties.

Facilitate Client Focus on Own Daily Life Adjustment

Overall, it is important to help college students with ADHD to identify the areas of daily living that they would like to improve. After reviewing the above background information with the client, we encourage the therapist to engage in a discussion with the client to determine areas of daily living that need improvement. You should take some time to do this (~10–15 min). An interactive approach that you could use is to ask you client if they recognize any difficulties in their own life in these areas (e.g., keeping track of finances, problems in the workplace) and then mention that these are areas that adults with ADHD have been shown to have difficulty with (you could also reverse this order of discussion). It might also help to probe for other things that the person sees as daily living tasks that their ADHD has gotten in the way of. The following example (see Dialogue 1) and discussion prompts will help to identify areas to target in Session 2 of this skill.

Dialogue 1

Therapist: As we just reviewed, many college students with ADHD have difficulties with daily life activities. Just as we have talked about strategies for managing other problem areas, like academics, relationships, or physical health, in the next session, we will also review some strategies for managing daily life activities. But, first we need to identify which, if any, areas of daily living are difficult for you. Does this plan sound okay?

Client:	*Yes. I know I struggle in almost all the areas you talked about, but making changes is so hard. Sometimes I try to make a change, but it just doesn't stick.*
Therapist:	*I hear what you are saying. I want you to know that if you decide to try again with making changes in any of these areas, with my support, the skills you have already learned in this program, and the strategies we will review next time, you might be more successful than in the past. Would it be okay if we talked through the difficulties you are having in each of the areas of daily living?*
Client:	*Yes, that works for me.*

The therapist should begin a discussion of areas of daily living. Examples of the types of questions to ask for each area are included below. A Daily Living Worksheet is provided in Appendix A that may help you to work with your client(s) on this.

Living Space, Home Workspace, and Laundry

- What is your living space like?
- Is your living space tidy or messy?
- Do you have trouble finding your car keys, wallet, or cell phone?
- Do you have a home workspace, like where you keep materials for school, bills, and personal documents? This could be a desk area or a separate room in your house.
- How do you organize these materials? Can you find materials when you need to?
- How often do you do laundry? Do you usually run out of clean clothes?
- How often do you clean your living space, such as vacuuming, dusting, emptying trash cans, and cleaning bathrooms and kitchens?
- How often do you wash your dishes? Do you often run out of clean dishes?
- Do you have specific concerns about your daily living space, laundry, or home workspace?

Grocery Shopping and Food Preparation

- What are your grocery shopping and food preparation strategies?
- How often do you shop for groceries?
- Do you make a list before you grocery shop?
- Do you go to multiple stores or just one?
- Do you order groceries or household goods online?
- Do you prepare food at home?
- Do you plan your food preparation for the week?

- Do you eat the groceries that you purchase (e.g., fruits and salad fixings) before they go bad?

Finances

- Do you manage your own finances, like paying bills, keeping up with account balances, and filing your tax return?
- What are your strategies for managing your finances?
- Do you often run out of money or overspend?
- Do you keep up with your account balances?
- Do you use online banking or an app to manage bill paying/accounts?
- Do you often run out of money before the end of the month?
- Do your parents get frustrated because you end up asking for more money?
- Do you manage your taxes or do your parents do this for you?
- Do you pay your credit card in full at the end of every month?
- Do you have credit card debt?

Errands and Appointments

- Do you have difficulties managing errands and appointments (e.g., doctor and dentist appointments, haircut appointments, and things like renewing driver's license)?
- Do you have a calendar system for keeping track of appointments?
- Do you see a dentist, eye doctor, and/or PCP at least once a year?
- Do you make these appointments in your college town or in your home-town?
- Do your parents help you with these tasks?
- Do you wait longer than you would like between haircuts and dentist appointments?
- Do you have a car? Do you remember to update your registration before your tags expire each year?

Making Travel and/or Social Plans

- Do you make your own travel plans for winter, spring, and summer breaks or do your parents help with this?
- If you make your own plans, do you often wait too long to make these plans so that the trip ends up being more stressful (e.g., figuring out which day you will fly or drive home for winter break, finding summer storage for your belongings, putting a down payment on a spring break trip that you want to take with your friends)?
- Do you miss out on social opportunities because you don't plan far enough ahead (e.g., by the time you ask your friends to do something on the weekend, they already have other plans)?

Work-related Issues

- Do you have or wish to have a part-time job?
- Have you had difficulty getting or keeping a job in the past? If so, what aspects were difficult for you?
- Do you have trouble getting to a job on time? Doing the assigned duties? Getting along with your manager or co-workers?
- Do you forget to ask for time off far enough in advance?
- Are you frequently late for work?

After collecting information about problems in daily living, work with the client to determine which area or areas they would like to focus on in the following session. We recommend that you help the client choose 1–3 areas to work on at one time. If the client does not appear to be motivated to make changes in a particular area even though problems are clearly identified, you may wish to try some motivational interviewing to help solidify reasons for making changes and identify goals.

Discuss Homework and Scheduling Next Session

For homework this week, clients should be asked to identify 1–3 areas on which they would like to work. During the week, clients should self-monitor these behaviors and observe their feelings, thoughts, and actions around those tasks. This information will be used to inform change efforts in the next section. Make sure to schedule the next session before the client departs.

References

Barkley, R.A., Fischer, M., Smallish, L., & Fletcher, K. (2002). The persistence of attention-deficit/hyperactivity disorder into young adulthood as a function of reporting source and definition of disorder. *Journal of Abnormal Psychology*, *111*(2), 279–289.

Fuermaier, A.B., Tucha, L., Butzbach, M., Weisbrod, M., Aschenbrenner, S., & Tucha, O. (2021). ADHD at the workplace: ADHD symptoms, diagnostic status, and work-related functioning. *Journal of Neural Transmission*, *128*, 1021–1031. 10.1007/s00702-021-02309-z

Holst, Y., & Thorell, L.B. (2020). Functional impairments among adults with ADHD: A comparison with adults with other psychiatric disorders and links to executive deficits. *Applied Neuropsychology Adult*, *27*(3), 243–255. 10.1080/23279095.2018.1532429

Session 2: Strategies for Effectively Managing Important Life Activities

Corresponds to Module 6.1–6.3 of the
Thriving in College Student Workbook

Session Outline

1 Check-in with client(s)
2 Set agenda
3 Orient clients to strategies that address their daily living concerns
4 Discuss homework
5 Schedule the next session

Session Organization

Administration Format

Session 2 (and any subsequent sessions in this module) should be administered in an individual format since each client will have identified the specific areas that they would like to work on. If the student would like to work on several of the areas, you may need two or more sessions to cover strategies and have the client select which they would like to use.

Materials Needed

Attending students should have a notebook or pad of paper to take notes. It may be helpful for the therapist to have some organizing visual materials, either in a projected PowerPoint, flipchart, or handouts. A copy of the Daily Living Strategies handout (see Appendix A) would likely be helpful.

Session Content

Check-in with Client

It is unlikely that this will be the first technique or content-heavy session that a client has done with you. Check-in time can be used to solicit brief discussion, or simply to see how things are going and build rapport. If this session is the first meeting with clients, check-in might focus more on feelings and expectations about therapy. In any event, aim for this to be brief (< 5 minutes), encouraging

DOI: 10.4324/9781003149590-28

for any additional discussion of this sort to be postponed until after the session content is completed. See therapist-client check-in dialogue example in Skill 1: Session 1 as a model for this interaction, if needed. We also recommend having your client complete the *Progress Tracker* (see Appendix B), and briefly touching base on any declines or improvements in school functioning.

Set Agenda

Introduce the agenda for this session to the client (see Session Outline). Again, it may be helpful to have a visual aid to refer to, such as a flip chart or projected PowerPoint slide or printed handout. At this time, it also might also be helpful to remind clients to write notes regarding important points in a therapy notebook. Settingthe agenda should be speedily completed (< 2 minutes). See therapist-client agenda-setting dialogue example in Skill 1: Session 1 as a model, if needed.

Orient Clients to Strategies that Address their daily Living Concerns

In the following text, we provide numerous ideas for clients to choose from to help them reach their goals in each of these daily life activities. Depending on the areas that your client has identified some maladjustment in, discuss these strategies as potential starting points for improvement. We recommend that you also discuss the applicability of previously learned OTMP and cognitive strategies to improving the management of daily life activities. Clients do not need to endorse or adopt all possible strategies in an area, but you may want to encourage them to try more than one as a start. A Daily Living Strategies handout is available in Appendix A should you wish to give the specific recommendations mentioned later directly to your client(s).

Strategies for Keeping a Clean Living Space and Doing Laundry

- Set weekly times in your calendar to: (a) straighten your living space; (b) clean your living space; (c) do your laundry
- Ask your roommates to agree to a standard time for all of you to straighten and clean together (i.e., to be your accountability partner … and you can be theirs!)
- Pair something enjoyable with each of these tasks (e.g., we always clean our apartment on Sundays before we go out for brunch or dinner; I always do my laundry on Saturdays while watching Netflix)
- When doing laundry, set alarms to remind yourself to start a load in the washing machine, transfer a load from washer to dryer, take laundry out of dryer, fold, put away

- For laundry, make a chart of any special washing instructions for your clothing items and post near your washer and dryer or keep with the supplies you take to the laundromat
- Establish a place where you always keep important items, like your keys and wallet (e.g., a basket or hook right inside your door)
- Consider using an electronic tracking device system (e.g., Tile, Apple AIRTAG) to keep track of frequently misplaced items like your phone and keys
- Do your dishes at the end of each day instead of letting them pile up over several days; listen to your favorite music or podcast while you do your dishes, or save dessert until after you have done your dishes
- Reward yourself for successes in these areas. For example, a week of doing your dishes daily = a movie night with friends
- Use time cracks (remember these?!) to clean or straighten your living space
- Do one cleaning task daily rather than saving them to do all at once so it is less of a burdensome task (e.g., Monday is dusting, Tuesday is vacuuming, Wednesday is cleaning the bathroom, etc.)
- If you have the money, consider hiring a cleaning service for a one-time deep clean to get you started.

Strategies for Organizing a Home Workspace or Office

- Set weekly times in your calendar for organizing home workspace or office
- Have a daily routine for this task (e.g., I always straighten my desk before I start my homework)
- Make sure you have an area for doing homework that isn't used for other things (e.g., don't put your clean laundry on your desk where you need to do your homework)
- Make sure you have materials in your homework area that you might need so that you can be more efficient when you sit down to work (e.g., paper, pens, laptop charger cord, calculator)
- As a general rule of thumb, don't turn one task into two (e.g., after you fold your laundry, put it away immediately rather than putting it on your desk where you will have to move it before you can start your homework)
- Consider using a filing system (a drawer or even a banker's box) to organize important documents, like your apartment rental agreement, passport, academic documents, instructions booklets for TV, etc.
- Organize your electronic documents into folders and subfolders on your computer

Strategies for Successful Grocery Shopping and Food Preparation

- Set weekly times in your calendar for grocery shopping and food preparation

- Try to limit grocery shopping to 1–3 times per week by planning for a few days in advance
- Recruit roommates, friends, or significant others as accountability partners
- Remember that you can gain efficiency and time by preparing meals that are big enough to have leftovers. Consider starting with one thing that you can make on the weekend and then eat throughout the week (e.g., make a pan of lasagna and divvy it into single serving size containers that you can eat throughout the week)
- Make a grocery list before you go to the store; organize by aisle if you always shop at the same store to avoid forgetting items and going back and forth
- Begin with a base list of things you need each week (e.g., milk, bread, coffee) and add to it things that are specific to that week
- Lean on electronic helpers. Some online recipes will add items to a grocery list for you, and some grocery stores will let you make a list online that you can re-use weekly
- Buy pre-prepped foods to make food preparation easier (e.g., pre-washed salad greens, pre-chopped veggies, pre-cooked meats). Note: These are not the same sort of thing as ready-to-go meals (e.g., frozen dishes), which tend to not have as much nutritional value and tend not to be good deals, moneywise
- Look for "meal of the day" or "meal of the week" specials at your grocery store. Some stores will have a recipe card and all the ingredients needed at the front. Others will have meal specials (e.g., a rotisserie chicken and two sides) that are pretty healthy and easy to prepare

Strategies for Managing your Finances

- Put bill paying and reviewing your finances on your calendar monthly
- Always pay your credit card bill in full or use a debit card instead to avoid paying interest
- Review your bank and credit card statements once a month; use the online banking feature which often includes an app where you can access account information quickly and easily
- Set up automatic bill payment through your bank or utility companies for recurrent and predictable expenses (e.g., cell phone bill, car insurance, rent)
- If you have the money, pay several months ahead on the bills at one time
- If you have trouble following through on these tasks, find an accountability partner, such as a significant other or parent, who might be willing to physically sit with you (in-person or by Zoom) while you complete these tasks
- If your parents provide you with money every month and you often run out before the next installment, ask your parents to send you money weekly rather than monthly
- Save up for big expenses, like a vacation, by setting aside a little money into a savings account each month. You can also set this up to automatically occur through your bank

Strategies for Completing Errands and Appointments

- Put appointments on your calendar, set a reminder or notification 1 week and 1 day before the appointment
- Pick a month (e.g., August right before school starts, December/January between semesters) when you schedule your yearly doctor and dentist appointments; put calling to schedule these appointments on your calendar for two months before the month in which you'd like to have the appointment
- When you are at an appointment (e.g., haircut), schedule your next appointment and immediately put it on your calendar

Managing Travel or Social Plans

- Put your travel dates on your calendar at the start of the semester
- Let your family members and/or significant other know your dates/plans
- Determine whether you need to book flights or make storage arrangements and put those tasks on your to-list if needed
- Early in the week, think about plans you would like to make for the weekend (e.g., go to a football game or party with friends, meet with a study group, hike or bike with friends)
- Decide when you would like to contact your friends about these plans and either send them a text or chat message or put it on your list of things to do for a specific day of the week

Discuss Homework and Schedule Next Session

Last session, clients identified 1–3 areas that they wanted to work on improving. They were also asked to self-monitor these behaviors and self-observe their feelings, thoughts, and actions around those tasks. First, you should discuss which areas they identified and then ask what they observed over the course of the week. Next, ask your client which of the aforementioned strategies they would like to try going forward in the areas they identified. Finally, be sure to schedule the next session (if needed) before the client departs.

Session 3: Succeeding at Work and Crafting a Career

Corresponds to Module 6.4 of the *Thriving in College* Student Workbook

Session Outline

1 Check-in with client(s)
2 Set agenda
3 Targeting and leveraging key job skills
4 Apply previously learned skills to the workplace
5 Career exploration and planning
6 Accommodations on the job
7 Discuss homework
8 Schedule next session

Session Organization

This session is recommended for clients who would like support regarding succeeding in a part-time job and planning for their career. Because work is a key area of impairment for adults with ADHD with long-term consequences (Barkley, 2015), this stand-alone session focuses on applying skills in the workplace, considering career directions, and understanding the use of accommodations on the job.

Administration Format

Session 3 can be administered in a group or individual format; however, a group format may be better suited, since the session involves discussion of career aspirations and experiences that multiple clients could benefit from.

Materials Needed

The therapist should have a whiteboard, flipchart, or a projected digital document to capture group ideas and/or present material.

DOI: 10.4324/9781003149590-29

- A list of or handout with "take-home messages" regarding the session's content as well as instructions/goals for at-home work prior to the next session is also useful to have for the client to refer to later.

Session Content

Check-in with Client(s)

It is unlikely that this will be the first technique or content-heavy session that a client has done with you. Check-in time can be used to solicit brief discussion about homework or issues that the client is dealing with currently, or simply to see how things are going and strengthen rapport. We also recommend having your client complete the *Progress Tracker* (see Appendix B), and briefly touching base on any declines or improvements in school functioning.

Set Agenda

Introduce the agenda for this session to the client (see Session Outline). It is helpful to have a visual aid to refer to, such as a flip chart or projected Powerpoint slide or printed handout. At this time it might also be helpful to remind clients to take notes regarding important points in a therapy notebook. Setting the agenda should be speedily completed (< 2 minutes). See therapist-client agenda-setting dialogue example in Skill 1: Session 1 as a model, if needed.

Targeting and Leveraging Key Job Skills

The first activity in this session focuses on helping clients to identify the key skills they need to be successful in the workplace. This is relevant both for college students who are currently employed and for those who are looking forward to a job in the future. Improving workplace-related skills is not only about cultivating positive relationships, but it is also about being a dependable employee and team player. These represent first steps toward establishing trust, confidence, and friendliness with supervisors and fellow employees. Further, having a satisfactory employment skill set is something that predicts retention and advancement in a job.

A survey of employers by the Collegiate Employment Research Institute identified six key behaviors that resulted in recent college-graduate hires being fired and seven qualities that were associated with hires being given promotions and new assignments in the company (Gardner, 2007). These are noted in Table 1 and Table 2. One challenge in trying to help clients develop and demonstrate these desirable qualities is the somewhat vague nature of these qualities; in other words, some of these qualities are difficult to operationalize

Table 1 Summary of reasons new college hires are retained based on employer surveys (Gardner, 2007)

How to Keep Your Job	*Strength?*	*Weakness?*	*Priority for Change*
Behave ethically			
Display motivation and work ethic			
Use technology appropriately			
Follow instructions			
Show up for work and show up on time			
Complete assignments by their deadlines			

Table 2 Summary of reasons new college hires are promoted based on employer surveys (Gardner, 2007)

How to Advance in Your Job	*Strength?*	*Weakness?*	*Priority for Change*
Take initiative to complete tasks and solve problems			
Self-regulate and self-motivate			
Display a positive and flexible attitude			
Show commitment and passion for the work			
Motivate others toward common goals			
Communicate clearly and persuasively			
Demonstrate technical knowledge and competence			

(e.g., "self-regulate") while others are more concrete (e.g., "complete assignments by their deadlines"). To aid in setting specific and measurable workplace goals, present the lists to the client and discuss the following:

- Beginning with Table 1, "How to Keep Your Job," **discuss what it would "look like"** to behave in line with each desirable quality. In other words, what specifically would the client's employer and fellow employees observe them doing (or NOT doing)?
- Which of these does the client believe are **current strengths** for them in the workplace?
- Which of these behaviors and skills is the **most in need of development** for them (i.e., represents a weakness)?
- Which skill(s) would they like to commit to working on in the next week (i.e., is a priority for change)?

After focusing on skills that can get employees into trouble in the workplace, pivot to a strengths-oriented discussion of behaviors that employers identified as associated with promotions, presented in Table 2, repeating the aforementioned steps to identify one or more priorities for change.

Next, discuss with the client which OTMP, cognitive, communication or other skills previously learned during the program (e.g., at-work task prioritization) that could be applied to their priority area for change in the workplace, and help the client develop a homework assignment that enacts this plan using Table 3. In particular, look for ways that clients might leverage or enhance their strengths in the workplace in the process of dealing with their weaknesses.

Table 3 Workplace Skills to Develop

Skill to Develop	Actions I'll Take This Week	Tools and Strategies I know that can help	Added to Task List / Calendar? (check)

For example:

1 Paulo identifies taking initiative for tasks as a strength, but admits that he often does not follow through on these commitments by the deadlines that his employer lays out. He and his therapist discuss adding work-related deadlines to his calendar and not taking on any new voluntary tasks at work until all prior tasks are completed.

2 Angie admits that she is not always truthful about the time she arrives at work because she is worried about the consequences of showing up late, which has been a chronic problem for her. She also realizes she is not communicating clearly with her employer about how her job is fitting in with her other commitments. With the help of her therapist, Angie decides to have a meeting with her supervisor to discuss her current number of hours and to share with her supervisor the strategies she will start using to help her get to work on time such as use of pre-programmed alarms in her phone. Above all, Angie wants to commit to being honest with her boss in the future.

3 Greg loves to communicate with and help people at his front-facing, customer-oriented job. However, he realizes he struggles to stay off his phone, which is prohibited at work, and has gotten reprimanded twice for this behavior. With his therapist, Greg decides that he will turn his phone off and put it in a drawer in another room during his work shifts. He also plans to ask his supervisor if there are other work tasks he could do at the front desk between working with customers, which he thinks could reduce his boredom and show initiative to help out.

We cannot anticipate all of the challenges and solutions that might be possible for clients in the workplace; instead, we invite you to tailor your approach to each clients' situation and strengths to arrive at a unique behavioral solution. Importantly, as is the case with any new behavior in this program, focus on helping the client implement the new skill by setting a specific goal, adding motivational and accountability enhancements, and following up on the homework assignment during the next session.

Career Exploration and Planning

Emphasize the Importance of Career "Fit" for People with ADHD

Educate the client about the importance of good career "fit" for adults with ADHD, including the following:

- Many adults with ADHD report that the severity of their symptoms depends on context and that they can reduce the impact of their symptoms by choosing work environments that are a better fit (Lasky et al., 2016). For instance, being a sports trainer (hands-on work, not a desk job) may be a good, natural fit for someone with ADHD.
- On the other hand, people with ADHD who choose careers that are a poor fit with their ADHD – for example, careers that require monotonous work, precise attention to detail, or lots of paperwork – may end up regretting their choices (Lasky et al., 2016). For example, it may not be the best fit for someone with ADHD to be an airline pilot (given inherent and severe possible consequences of inattention).
- In interviewing 125 young adults diagnosed with ADHD as children, Lasky and colleagues (2016) found that many preferred work that was:
  - Stressful and challenging
  - Novel and required multitasking
  - Busy and fast-paced
  - Physically demanding or hands-on
  - Intrinsically interesting
- Strong interest in the work task may be especially important to maintaining motivation for workers with ADHD (Lyhne et al., 2021). Some adults with ADHD reported that finding a job that was intensely interesting to them reduced their problems with focus and follow-through (Lasky et al., 2016).
- People with ADHD may be drawn to entrepreneurship and start-up ventures; however, untreated symptoms may get in the way of persisting in running one's own business (Greidanus & Liao, 2021).

Discuss Client's Perceptions of What Careers Might Be a Good Fit

Briefly discuss with the client what kinds of jobs, tasks, or career tracks they think might be a good fit for them. What kinds of work do they enjoy? Are there any activities that have kept them motivated and interested long-term? The goal here is simply to introduce and normalize the idea of goodness-of-fit, not to identify final career directions. Invite the client to think expansively and creatively about what their work life could look like in the future. You might suggest that the client review lists of possible careers online or even complete a brief online survey to begin to think about what types of careers might work best (e.g., https://www.123test.com/career-test/).

Discuss Barriers to Finding a Good-Fit Career

College students are often influenced in their career choices by factors that can impede their ability to choose a best-fit career, such as perceptions of prestige or financial security or the expectations of their parents, real or perceived. Briefly discuss with the client what barriers they perceive to finding a good-fitting career. Emphasize and validate their perceptions of these barriers, but express optimism that there may still be ways to consider career fit even within necessary constraints.

Dialogue 1

Therapist: *Okay, you mentioned that your favorite job you've had so far was working as a skiing instructor during your winter breaks. Tell me more about that. What did you like about it?*

Client: *Well, obviously I really like skiing, but I think my favorite thing is that I really get to help people improve and learn to love the sport. There's always something you can improve on as a skier and every client has different needs in terms of what they should learn next and what approach is going to work best to help them learn it. No two days are ever the same out there!*

Therapist: *Cool, so it sounds like the work itself is interesting to you, which can be especially important to keeping you engaged and motivated. How does your ADHD affect you when you're doing that job?*

Client: *I guess my biggest problems are pretty typical to what I experience in college – showing up on time and keeping my schedule straight. But once I'm there, I'm "on" and the time just flies by. Also, I work with some great people and that keeps me in it, too.*

Therapist: *Okay, so I think maybe this is giving us some clues about the kind of work might be most engaging for you.*

Client:	*Yeah, right. I can't be a ski instructor for the rest of my life!*
Therapist:	*Why not?*
Client:	*Money, for one, it doesn't pay enough. And my dad would say it was a waste of my college degree to just be a ski bum. That's why he wants me to declare an accounting major. It's the fastest track to a secure, good-paying job of all the majors, really. I'll probably be recruited by a firm before I even graduate.*
Therapist:	*Definitely makes sense that you need to find a career where you can support yourself, I get that! I guess I just want to invite you to be curious about what kinds of work and work settings fit best with your strengths. Like we talked about, finding a good fit between you and your work is important for everyone, but it might be even **more** important for people with ADHD. Do you have a sense of what the day-to-day of being an accountant might look like?*
Client:	*.... I don't know, actually. I assume working on spreadsheets at a desk a lot? I hadn't really thought about it much.*
Therapist:	*Makes sense to me! It's hard to know what a job is like until you actually do it. Do you think you'd be willing to make an appointment at career services to learn more about what accounting is like and maybe also get some more information about your career interests? You might even be able to shadow or get mentored by an accountant to get some first-hand information.*

Plan Steps to Access Career Services on Campus

The career services office at the student's institution should be equipped to provide formal assessment of the career values and interests that can help students with ADHD identify career trajectories they may want to explore (Dipeolu, 2011). Work with the client in session to set up an appointment with the appropriate office on their campus and add the appointment to their calendar, setting attendance at the appointment as a homework assignment for the week.

Considering Accommodations on the Job

Provide Psychoeducation and Coaching About Workplace Accommodations

Some clients may benefit from workplace accommodations to aid in managing the impact of ADHD on the job, but few may be aware that they can request accommodations or how to approach this process. Discuss the basics of workplace accommodation with the client, presented later. If you have not previously discussed academic accommodations, it may be useful to present this information first (see Skill 2, Session 2, Table 1) to provide context.

The Americans with Disabilities Act (ADA) and the Rehabilitation Act of 1973 prohibit discrimination against people with disabilities in the workplace. ADA offers the most expansive protections and applies to private employers with 15 or more employees, state and local governments, and "places of public accommodation," which encompasses many workplaces including institutions of higher education (CHADD National Resource Center on ADHD, 2021). As is the case for the classroom, the ADA requires that reasonable accommodations be made for people with disabilities who are "otherwise qualified" to ensure equal access to the workplace. Employees must disclose their disability status – although they need not disclose the specific diagnosis – to the employer and proactively make the request for accommodation. This is often a daunting step for clients and they will want to consider carefully the benefits and, unfortunately, potential costs of disclosure.

If your client would like to discuss how to decide upon and request workplace accommodations, ask them to identify work-related situations where their ADHD symptoms get in the way and ideas for support they might obtain to lower these barriers. Importantly, the accommodation should not create an undue hardship for the employer, although this can be hard to define (ADA National Network, 2018). We have provided a Reasonable Accommodations in the Workplace handout in Appendix A that may be a helpful reference to you and your client(s).

Finally, if relevant, work with the client to plan out how they will request the accommodation, employing communication skill strategies such as role-playing, if appropriate. Clients may wish to consider framing their requests from a position of strength, emphasizing what the accommodation will help them accomplish, rather than focusing on the disability itself (CHADD National Resource Center on ADHD, 2021).

Discuss Homework and Schedule Next Session

Review the goals and tasks for the next week that have emerged from this session including actions to apply previously learned skills in the workplace, any plans to obtain career counseling or services, and plans for requesting workplace accommodations. Make sure that the client has put the action items in their task list and any relevant appointments into their calendar. If needed at this point, schedule the next session to meet with the client before the client departs.

References

ADA National Network. (2018). Reasonable accommodations in the workplace. *ADA National Network*. https://adata.org/factsheet/reasonable-accommodations-workplace

Barkley, R.A. (Ed.) (2015). Educational, occupational, dating and marital, and financial impairments in adults with ADHD. In *Attention-deficit hyperactivity disorder: A handbook for diagnosis and treatment*. (pp. 314–342). The Guilford Press.

CHADD National Resource Center on ADHD. (2021). For adults: Workplace issues. *CHADD.Org*. https://chadd.org/for-adults/workplace-issues/

Dipeolu, A.O. (2011). College students with ADHD: Prescriptive concepts for best practices in career development. *Journal of Career Development, 38*(5), 408–427. 10.1177/0894845310378749

Gardner, P. (2007). Moving up or moving out of the company? *Collegiate Employment Research Institute*, Michigan State University.

Greidanus, N.S., & Liao, C. (2021). Toward a coping-dueling-fit theory of the ADHD-entrepreneurship relationship: Treatment's influence on business venturing, performance, and persistence. *Journal of Business Venturing, 36*(2), 106087. 10.1016/j.jbusvent.2020.106087

Lasky, A.K., Weisner, T.S., Jensen, P.S., Hinshaw, S.P., Hechtman, L., Arnold, L.E., W. Murray, D., & Swanson, J.M. (2016). ADHD in context: Young adults' reports of the impact of occupational environment on the manifestation of ADHD. *Social Science & Medicine, 161*, 160–168. 10.1016/j.socscimed.2016.06.003

Lyhne, C.N., Pedersen, P., Nielsen, C.V., & Bjerrum, M.B. (2021). Needs for occupational assistance among young adults with ADHD to deal with executive impairments and promote occupational participation—A qualitative study. *Nordic Journal of Psychiatry, 75*(5), 362–369. 10.1080/08039488.2020.1862911

Appendix A: Handouts for Clients

Contents:

231 ... Task Prioritization Handout (OTMP, Skill 1 – Session 3)

232 ... Academic Skills Practice (Professional Learner, Skill 2 – Session 1)

233 ... Academic Skills Practice Planning (Professional Learner, Skill 2 – Session 1)

234 ... Self-Monitoring Form (Thinking and Responding Differently, Skill 3 – Session 1)

235 ... Daily Thought Record Ver. 1 (Thinking & Responding Differently, Skill 3 – Session 2)

236 ... Daily Thought Record Ver. 2 (Thinking & Responding Differently, Skill 3 – Session 3)

237 ... Healthy Lifestyles: Identifying Your Target (Taking Good Care of Yourself, Skill 4 – Session 2)

238 ... Improving Sleep (Taking Good Care of Yourself, Skill 4 – Session 3)

240 ... Improving Diet (Taking Good Care of Yourself, Skill 4 – Session 3)

241 ... Improving Physical Activity (Taking Good Care of Yourself, Skill 4 – Session 3)

242 ... Moderating Substance Use (Taking Good Care of Yourself, Skill 4 – Session 3)

243 ... Moderating Technology Use (Taking Good Care of Yourself, Skill 4 – Session 3)

244 ... Driving Safely (Taking Good Care of Yourself, Skill 4 – Session 3)

245 ... Relational Worksheet (Being Successful in Relationships, Skill 5 – Session 2)

247 ... Daily Living Worksheet ("Adulting," Skill 6 – Session 1)

251 ... Daily Living Strategies ("Adulting," Skill 6 – Session 2)

254 ... Reasonable Accommodations in the Workplace ("Adulting," Skill 6 – Session 3)

Task Prioritization Worksheet

Urgent and Important:	Not Urgent but Important
1.	1.
2.	2.
3.	3.
4.	4.
5.	5.
Urgent but Not as Important:	**Not as Urgent and Not as Important:**
1.	1.
2.	2.
3.	3.
4.	4.
5.	5.

Academic Skills Practice

Choose at least two skills you would like to practice in the coming week from the choices below.

Strategies to Increase Focus (Stay "In the Zone")

- Create a low-distraction study environment using the handout provided
- Practice using the Pomodoro Technique with an app or physical timer

Effective Learning and Memory Strategies

- Practice self-testing when studying for upcoming tests or quizzes
- Schedule a few spread out study sessions in advance of a test or quiz (distributed practice)
- Formulate and practice some new mnemonics for tough concepts in classes

Note-Taking Strategies

- Practice the two-column note taking method in your classes

Getting Help from Professors

- Review the following resources for your classes: syllabus, learning management system, instructions for upcoming assignments
- Attend your professors' office hours
- Practice writing an effective email to an instructor

Getting Help from Peers

- Write to a peer to ask for notes from a missed class
- Set up a study group with peers
- Practice clear communication with peers on a group project

Academic Skills Practice Planning

Skill to Practice	What, specifically, will you do to practice? (Add to task list)	When will you do this? (Add to calendar)
(if needed)		

Self-Monitoring Form

Instructions: In several different moments over the next few days, notice what is going on in the environment and inside of you and record it below.

What do I SEE?	What do I HEAR?	What do I SMELL/TASTE?	What do I feel ON MY SKIN?	What do I feel INSIDE MY BODY?	How is my body MOVING?	What THOUGHTS do I have?

Daily Thought Record V. 1 (Noticing your Patterns)

Instructions: For at least one situation per day, complete the table below. Choose situations where your ADHD symptoms contributed to problems for you. Alternatively, you can choose situations where you experienced strong emotions.

Situation – when and where?	Feelings	Thoughts	Action	Why was this action problematic?

Daily Thought Record Ver. 2 (Practicing New Responses)

Instructions: For at least one situation per day, complete the table below. Choose situations where your ADHD symptoms contributed to problems for you. Alternatively, you can choose situations where you experienced strong emotions.

Situation – when and where?	Feelings	Thoughts	Action	Why was this action problematic?	Alternative thoughts and actions

Healthy Lifestyles: Identifying Your Targets

Think about each of the six major health areas below and write a few sentences about how you are doing with each of these lifestyle areas. **What is going well and what is causing problems** for you in your life right now?

Thoughts about my sleep habits:

Thoughts about my eating habits and nutrition:

Thoughts about my exercise and level of physical activity:

Thoughts about my use of alcohol, nicotine, and other drugs:

Thoughts about my use of technology:

Thoughts about my driving:

Now, based on what you wrote, answer the following questions:

Which lifestyle area is currently **causing the most problems** in your life (check one)?

❐ Sleep   ❐ Eating and Nutrition   ❐ Exercise   ❐ Substance Use   ❐ Tech Use   ❐ Driving

Which lifestyle area are you currently **managing the most effectively** (check one)?

❐ Sleep   ❐ Eating and Nutrition   ❐ Exercise   ❐ Substance Use   ❐ Tech Use   ❐ Driving

Which lifestyle area do you feel **most capable of changing right now** (check one)?

❐ Sleep   ❐ Eating and Nutrition   ❐ Exercise   ❐ Substance Use   ❐ Tech Use   ❐ Driving

Looking back on your answers, which area **would you like to commit to working on right now**? Remember, it is okay to commit to *small changes* to start!

I'll commit to working on:_____

Improving Sleep

The following are suggestions that may help you to improve your sleep. Consider which one(s) you might be willing to try.

- Practice good sleep hygiene habits, which include:
    - Go to bed and wake up at roughly the same time each day, ideally also on weekends (though this is not possible for many college students). It is hard for your brain to adjust to different bedtimes each day.
    - Create a relaxing bedtime routine that does not involve a screen. Ideas include reading a book, listening to music, listening to an audio book, or taking a bath. There are smartphone apps like *Headspace* that include bedtime meditation, and other apps that will read you a bedtime story.
    - Try to stop using screens 30 minutes before bedtime.
    - Make sure your bedroom is cool (between 60 and 67 degrees is ideal).
    - Make sure your bedroom is quiet. Use earplugs or white noise if necessary.
    - Make sure that your bedroom is dark. It is hard to get good sleep with a TV on. Use blackout shades or other window coverings to keep the light out.
    - Finish eating meals 2–3 hours before bedtime. Stop using caffeine 4–6 hours before bedtime.
    - Alcohol and nicotine use can also disrupt sleep. For the best sleep, skip these close to bedtime.
    - Exercise regularly, but don't do vigorous exercise in the evening before bedtime.
    - Sleep on a mattress and pillows that are comfortable and supportive.
    - Don't go to bed unless you are sleepy. And, if you don't fall asleep within 20 minutes of going to bed, get up and do something relaxing.
- Schedule bedtime and wakeup time on your calendar.
- Set multiple alarms to help transition from highly engaging activities to prepare for sleep (e.g., one alarm to turn off screens, one alarm to turn off lights).
- Take your ADHD medications as prescribed. Prescription stimulant medications can disrupt sleep if taken too close to bedtime. Talk to your doctor if your ADHD medication is impacting your sleep.
- Limit your use of sleep aid medication. If you must use a sleep aid medication, melatonin and CBD are both generally safe and typically have no side effects. However, research evidence is limited for both of these sleep aids for insomnia, so it is best to speak with your doctor about options if you believe you need sleep aid medication.
- Seek treatment for co-occurring anxiety and depression as these conditions can also impact sleep in a negative way.

- Track your sleep and how it is impacting behavior. There are wearable devices (e.g., Apple Watch, FitBit) that will track your sleep for you and send the info to a smartphone app.
- Reward yourself for sticking to your new, healthy sleep habits, perhaps with new sheets, comfy PJs or bedroom slippers, or some bubble bath or lotion to use for relaxing before bedtime. Remember your strategies for rewarding yourself from the first few modules of this program.

Improving Diet

The following are suggestions that may help you to improve your diet. Consider which one(s) you might be willing to try.

- Determine your goals (e.g., eat healthier foods, eat more regularly, reduce emotional eating, lose weight, gain weight, improve blood chemistry).
- Eat several meals per day at regular times so that you have enough energy for your daily activities and do not go so long between meals that you tend to overeat as a result.
- Schedule meals on your calendar if you have difficulty remembering to eat or sticking to a regular eating schedule.
- Plan weekly meals and grocery shop once per week (e.g., Sunday) and schedule this time on your calendar.
- Prepare foods in advance (e.g., make a big pot of soup or a casserole that can be eaten for several meals during the week, prepare fruits and veggies so they can be quickly grabbed, make a big salad) and schedule this on your calendar.
- Prepare meals the night before if you will need to take with you or will not have time during your day (e.g., pack a lunch to take to campus).
- Buy healthy snacks and consider not bringing junk food into the house.
- Put some healthy snacks in your backpack in case you get hungry so that you are not tempted to purchase fast food when you were not planning on it or so that you do not get too hungry and overeat later.
- Keep a food diary or journal or use a smartphone app to track your food intake (e.g., *MyFitnessPal*, *MyPlate*).
- Plan a certain number of meals per week that you will eat out or get takeout and stick to your plans.
- Get familiar with recommended nutrition guidelines or visit a nutritionist if your student health service has one available.
- Buy a cookbook or subscribe to a recipe or meal planning site (e.g., Cooking Light, NYT Cooking).

Improving Physical Activity

The following are suggestions that may help you to be more physically active. Consider which one(s) you might be willing to try.

- Transportation

  ○ Walk or bike to work or on errands if feasible.
  ○ Take the stairs instead of the elevator.
  ○ Park further away from the store on purpose.
  ○ Use an activity or step tracker (e.g., FitBit, Garmin watch, Apple watch) with a smartphone app and set a daily steps goal.

- Exercise

  ○ Set a goal for how many times per week you would like to exercise. Let clients choose whether they want to focus on further, longer or faster.
  ○ Put exercise on your calendar and build into your day.
  ○ Consider whether you prefer working out alone or with others.
  ○ Find an accountability or work-out partner (e.g., make plans to workout with a friend to increase the likelihood that you will follow through). If your friend is at a different skill level you could have a plan to go together but not exercise together (e.g., swim at different speeds).
  ○ Consider joining a yoga studio or a gym. This can be helpful if you do not have a reliable workout partner because you might develop acquaintances or friendships at the gym and you might look forward to seeing these folks. You might also be more likely to go to an exercise class if you have already paid for it in advance.
  ○ Pick physical activities that you enjoy doing or that you find less aversive (e.g., if you dislike running because of the physical challenge, start with walking). Listen to music or an audiobook while exercising to make the experience more pleasant. Some researchers have referred to this as "temptation bundling" (e.g., Kirgios et al., 2020) and suggest only allowing yourself to listen to a particularly compelling book while exercising.
  ○ Join a club or a class to learn a new activity (e.g., take an introduction to cross-country skiing at outdoor program, attend a group workout class at campus recreation center)
  ○ Schedule exercise more frequently to plan for the inevitable times when it doesn't work out due to other more urgent tasks (e.g., if you want to exercise 3 times per week, then schedule 5 times knowing that you can skip 2 if the timing isn't working out).
  ○ Use a smartphone app that allows you to see what your friends and acquaintances are doing (e.g., Strava).
  ○ Reward yourself for meeting your daily steps goal or increasing your exercise sessions, perhaps with a new work-out outfit, tennis shoes, or a healthy smoothie.

Moderating Substance Use

The following are suggestions that may help you to use alcohol, if you choose to do so at all, in a safe way. Many of these can be helpful in moderating use of other substances, too. Consider which one(s) you might be willing to try.

- Track your use of alcohol and drugs. Set a goal of reducing use. Reward yourself for progress in this area, perhaps with a fun activity with friends that does not involve drinking or using drugs like playing paintball, going out for coffee, or taking a walk.
- There are several protective behavioral strategies that have been shown through research to be helpful to college students with ADHD for reducing alcohol use and the negative outcomes associated with use such as blacking out, being hungover, driving drunk, and missing class. Select the strategies that you think will be most helpful for you:
  - Set a limit on the number of drinks you will have in one drinking session. If you don't think you can keep track, put that many rubber bands on one wrist and each time you have a drink, remove a rubber band and put it in your pocket.
  - Mix and bring your own beverages. When what you bought is gone, stop drinking.
  - Avoid combining alcohol and marijuana. Combining substances can make you get more drunk/high and reduce your ability to make good decisions about limiting your use and staying safe.
  - Avoid pre-gaming or pre-partying.
  - Stop drinking at a predetermined time and drink water only after this time. This will also help you sleep better.
  - Eat a meal before or during drinking.
  - Avoid mixing different types of alcohol.
  - Drink slowly rather than gulp or chug. If you feel pressure to drink more, you can always pretend to take a sip now and then. You can also take your drink to the kitchen or bathroom or outside and pour some out.
  - Avoid trying to keep up or out drink others. Avoid drinking games.
  - Alternate alcoholic and nonalcoholic drinks. For every alcoholic drink you have, drink a glass of water. Or, put extra ice in your alcoholic drink to water it down.
  - Ask a friend to let you know when you have had enough to drink.
  - Only go out with people you know and trust and make sure you are with people who can take care of you if you drink too much.
  - Know where your drink has been at all times. Keep it in your hand. If you are at a party, bring your own drink container with a lid. These strategies will help to prevent others from "drugging" your drink.
  - Use a designated driver or a ride service like Uber.

Moderating Technology Use

The following are suggestions that may help you to use technology, like a mobile phone or the internet, in a reasonable way. Consider which one(s) you might be willing to try.

- Use airplane mode on your phone or turn off the internet on your computer to limit distractions when you are trying to be productive.
- Track your screen time using the settings on your phone or an app. Set a goal of reducing use. Reward yourself for progress in this area, perhaps with a fun activity with friends that does not involve technology like playing baseball, going out for coffee, or taking a walk.
- Set a limit on the number of minutes or hours you will spend per day engaging in a particular type of technology use (e.g., video gaming). Use phone timers or apps to remind yourself.
- Ask your partner, friend, or roommate to set shared goals regarding technology use (e.g., video gaming, Netflix) and try to hold each other accountable.
- Put your phone in the middle of the table when you are at a restaurant and ask your dining partners to do the same. You can make a game out of it by saying that whoever checks their phone first must pay the bill.
- Make a point of putting your phone in another room or in a location where you cannot easily access it (e.g., a drawer) while you are doing schoolwork or spending time with friends or use an app that doesn't allow you to use it while you are doing a Pomodoro (e.g., Forest or Flora).
- Carry a book with you so that you can read instead of watching YouTube or checking social media when you have a little down time between activities or must wait for a class or appointment.
- Use technology as a reward for completing other activities (e.g., when I finish this assignment, I will use my phone for 5 minutes; when I finish all my homework, I will play video games for an hour).

Driving Safely

The following are suggestions that may help you to drive in a safe manner. Consider which one(s) you might be willing to try.

- If you take stimulant medicine for your ADHD, take it regularly at the scheduled time. You will be a more attentive driver if you are taking your medication as prescribed.
- Schedule long driving trips early in the day when you are rested and alert. Take a break every 2 hours
- Set your phone to automatically go to do-not-disturb when you are driving. Leave your phone in the backseat or trunk while you are driving
- Adjust your radio or look up driving directions before you begin a drive, not during the drive
- Limit the number of passengers that you take in your car to reduce distractions while driving (e.g., driving 5 drunk friends to a party may be very distracting)
- Make a commitment not to drive after drinking or using drugs
- Consider taking a taxi, Uber, or Lyft instead of driving if there is a large group or anyone has been drinking or using drugs (if these services are not available where you are, call a friend)

Relational Worksheet

Situation (when? With who?)	**Behaviors** (check which you used)	**Result** (how did it end up?)
	__ **positive conflict resolution** *focusing on understanding each others' perspectives and potential solutions* __ **open communication** *staying positive and direct* __ **being a good listener** *reflecting content, using nonverbals* __ **reciprocity** *taking turns, checking in/emotions* __ **attention to wants/needs** *respecting/noticing partner's responses and personal needs*	
	__ **positive conflict resolution** *focusing on understanding each others' perspectives and potential solutions* __ **open communication** *staying positive and direct* __ **being a good listener** *reflecting content, using nonverbals* __ **reciprocity** *taking turns, checking in/emotions* __ **attention to wants/needs** *respecting/noticing partner's responses and personal needs*	
	__ **positive conflict resolution** *focusing on understanding each others' perspectives and potential solutions* __ **open communication** *staying positive and direct* __ **being a good listener** *reflecting content, using nonverbals* __ **reciprocity** *taking turns, checking in/emotions* __ **attention to wants/needs** *respecting/noticing partner's responses and personal needs*	

(Continued)

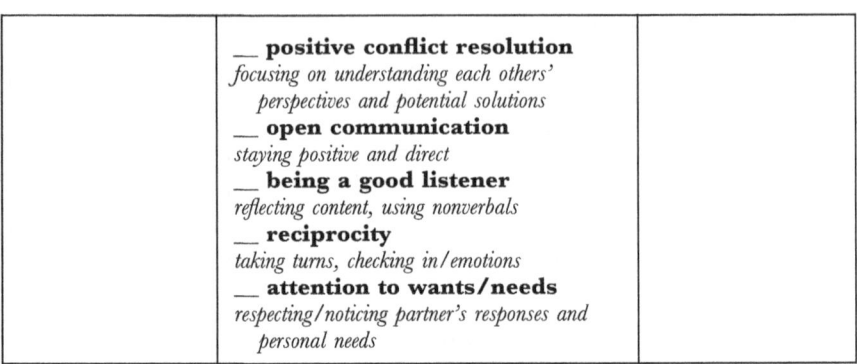

What Do You Take From These Observations? What Can You Do Differently Next Time?

_____

_____

Daily Living Worksheet

Put a check by any of the areas in bold below that you perceive you have some difficulty, and then answer any pertinent questions underneath. Keep this to consider in discussions with your therapist.

___ Living Space, Home Workspace, and Laundry

- What is your living space like?

- Is your living space tidy or messy?

- Do you have trouble finding your car keys, wallet, or cell phone?

- Do you have a home workspace, like where you keep materials for school, bills, and personal documents? This could be a desk area or a separate room in your house.

- How do you organize these materials? Can you find materials when you need to?

- How often do you do laundry? Do you usually run out of clean clothes?

- How often do you clean your living space, such as vacuuming, dusting, emptying trash cans, and cleaning bathrooms and kitchens?

- How often do you wash your dishes? Do you often run out of clean dishes?

- Do you have specific concerns about your daily living space, laundry, or home workspace?

___ Grocery Shopping and Food Preparation

- What are your grocery shopping and food preparation strategies?

- How often do you shop for groceries?

- Do you make a list before you grocery shop?

- Do you go to multiple stores or just one?

- Do you order groceries or household goods online?

- Do you prepare food at home?

- Do you plan your food preparation for the week?

- Do you eat the groceries that you purchase (e.g., fruits and salad fixings) before they go bad?

___ **Finances**
- Do you manage your own finances, like paying bills, keeping up with account balances, and filing your tax return?

- What are your strategies for managing your finances?

- Do you often run out of money or overspend?

- Do you keep up with your account balances?

- Do you use online banking or an app to manage bill paying/accounts?

- Do you often run out of money before the end of the month?

- Do your parents get frustrated because you end up asking for more money?

- Do you manage your taxes or do your parents do this for you?

- Do you pay your credit card in full at the end of every month?

- Do you have credit card debt?

___ Errands and Appointments

- Do you have difficulties managing errands and appointments (e.g., doctor and dentist appointments, haircut appointments, and things like renewing driver's license)?

- Do you have a calendar system for keeping track of appointments?

- Do you see a dentist, eye doctor, and/or PCP at least once a year?

- Do you make these appointments in your college town or in your hometown?

- Do your parents help you with these tasks?

- Do you wait longer than you would like between haircuts and dentist appointments?

- Do you have a car? Do you remember to update your registration before your tags expire each year?

___ Making Travel and/or Social Plans

- Do you make your own travel plans for winter, spring, and summer breaks or do your parents help with this?

- If you make your own plans, do you often wait too long to make these plans so that the trip ends up being more stressful (e.g., figuring out which day you will fly or drive home for winter break, finding summer storage for your belongings, putting a down payment on a spring break trip that you want to take with your friends)?

• Do you miss out on social opportunities because you don't plan far enough ahead (e.g., by the time you ask your friends to do something on the weekend, they already have other plans)?

___ Work-Related Issues

• Do you have or wish to have a part-time job?

• Have you had difficulty getting or keeping a job in the past? If so, what aspects were difficult for you?

• Do you have trouble getting to a job on time? Doing the assigned duties? Getting along with your manager or co-workers?

• Do you forget to ask for time off far enough in advance?

• Are you frequently late for work?

Daily Living Strategies

The following are a diverse set of strategies that can potentially help you to better handle daily living activities that get in the way or are difficult for you now. Circle or otherwise indicate behaviors below, based on discussion with your therapist, that you will try!

Strategies for *Keeping a Clean Living Space and doing Laundry*

- Set weekly times in your calendar to: (a) straighten your living space; (b) clean your living space; (c) do your laundry
- Ask your roommates to agree to a standard time for all of you to straighten and clean together (i.e., to be your accountability partner ... and you can be theirs!)
- Pair something enjoyable with each of these tasks (e.g., We always clean our apartment on Sundays before we go out for brunch or dinner; I always do my laundry on Saturdays while watching Netflix)
- When doing laundry, set alarms to remind yourself to start a load in the washing machine, transfer a load from washer to drying, take laundry out of dryer, fold, and fold and put away
- For laundry, make a chart of any special washing instructions for your clothing items and post near your washer and dryer or keep with the supplies you take to the laundromat
- Establish a place where you always keep important items, like your keys and wallet (e.g., a basket or hook right inside your door)
- Consider using an electronic tracking device system (e.g., Tile, Apple AIRTAG) to keep track of frequently misplaced items like your phone and keys
- Do your dishes at the end of each day instead of letting them pile up over several days; listen to your favorite music or podcast while you do your dishes, or save dessert until after you have done your dishes
- Reward yourself for successes in these areas. For example, a week of doing your dishes daily = a movie night with friends
- Use time cracks (remember these?!) to clean or straighten your living space
- Do one cleaning task daily rather than saving them to do all at once so it is less of a burdensome task (e.g., Monday is dusting, Tuesday is vacuuming, Wednesday is cleaning the bathroom, etc.)
- If you have the money, consider hiring a cleaning service for a one-time deep clean to get you started

Strategies for *Organizing a Home Workspace or Office*

- Set weekly times in your calendar for organizing home workspace or office
- Have a daily routine for this task (e.g., I always straighten my desk before I start my homework)

- Make sure you have an area for doing homework that isn't used for other things (e.g., Don't put your clean laundry on your desk where you need to do your homework)
- Make sure you have materials in your homework area that you might need so that you can be more efficient when you sit down to work (e.g., paper, pens, laptop charger cord, calculator)
- As a general rule of thumb, don't turn one task into two (e.g., after you fold your laundry, put it away immediately rather than putting it on your desk where you will have to move it before you can start your homework)
- Consider using a filing system (a drawer or even a banker's box) to organize important documents, like your apartment rental agreement, passport, academic documents, instructions booklets for TV, etc.
- Organize your electronic documents into folders and subfolders on your computer

Strategies for *Successful Grocery Shopping and Food Preparation*

- Set weekly times in your calendar for grocery shopping and food preparation
- Try to limit grocery shopping to 1–3 times per week by planning for a few days in advance
- Recruit roommates, friends, or significant others as accountability partners
- Remember that you can gain efficiency and time by preparing meals that are big enough to have leftovers. Consider starting with one thing that you can make on the weekend and then eat throughout the week (e.g., make a pan of lasagna and divvy it into single serving size containers that you can eat throughout the week)
- Make a grocery list before you go to the store; organize by aisle if you always shop at the same store to avoid forgetting items and going back and forth
- Begin with a base list of things you need each week (e.g., milk, bread, coffee) and add to it things that are specific to that week
- Lean on electronic helpers. Some online recipes will add items to a grocery list for you, and some grocery stores will let you make a list online that you can re-use weekly
- Buy pre-prepped foods to make food preparation easier (e.g., pre-washed salad greens, pre-chopped veggies, pre-cooked meats). Note: These are not the same sort of thing as ready-to-go meals (e.g., frozen dishes), which tend to not have as much nutritional value and tend not to be good deals, moneywise
- Look for "meal of the day" or "meal of the week" specials at your grocery store. Some stores will have a recipe card and all the ingredients needed at the front. Others will have meal specials (e.g., a rotisserie chicken and two sides) that are pretty healthy and easy to prepare

Strategies for *Managing your Finances*

- Put bill paying and reviewing your finances on your calendar monthly
- Always pay your credit card bill in full or use a debit card instead to avoid paying interest (see https://vimeo.com/199334296).
- Review your bank and credit card statements once a month; use the online banking feature which often includes an app where you can access account information quickly and easily
- Set up automatic bill payment through your bank or utility companies for recurrent and predictable expenses (e.g., cell phone bill, car insurance, rent)
- If you have the money, pay several months ahead of the bills at one time
- If you have trouble following through on these tasks, find an accountability partner, such as a significant other or parent, who might be willing to physically sit with you (in-person or by Zoom) while you complete these tasks
- If your parents provide you with money every month and you often run out before the next installment, ask your parents to send you money weekly rather than monthly
- Save up for big expenses, like a vacation, by setting aside a little money into a savings account each month. You can also set this up to automatically occur through your bank

Strategies for *Completing Errands and Appointments*

- Put appointments on your calendar, set a reminder or notification 1 week and 1 day before the appointment
- Pick a month (e.g., August right before school starts, Dec/Jan between semesters) when you schedule your yearly doctor and dentist appointments; put calling to schedule these appointments on your calendar for two months before the month in which you'd like to have the appointment
- When you are at an appointment (e.g., haircut), schedule your next appointment and immediately put it on your calendar

Strategies for *Managing Travel or Social Plans*

- Put your travel dates on your calendar at the start of the semester
- Let your family members and/or significant other know your dates/plans
- Determine whether you need to book flights or make storage arrangements and put those tasks on your to-list if needed
- Early in the week, think about plans you would like to make for the weekend (e.g., go to a football game or party with friends, meet with a study group, hike or bike with friends)
- Decide when you would like to contact your friends about these plans and either send them a text or chat message or put it on your list of things to do for a specific day of the week

Reasonable Accommodations in the Workplace

This fact sheet serves as a basic overview of reasonable accommodations in the workplace and includes some examples and a brief review of the reasonable accommodation process. This document has information that may be useful for employees, employers, human resources staff, and others. Because this is a very general, baseline document, more specific questions may be answered by the reader's local ADA Center.

Key Definitions

What is a Reasonable Accommodation?

A reasonable accommodation is any change to the application or hiring process, to the job, to the way the job is done, or the work environment that allows a person with a disability who is qualified for the job to perform the essential functions of that job and enjoy equal employment opportunities. Accommodations are considered "reasonable" if they do not create an undue hardship or a direct threat.

Who Is an "Individual with a Disability?"

An individual meets the Americans with Disabilities with Act definition act of "disability" that would qualify them for reasonable accommodations if they have "a physical or mental impairment that substantially limits one or more major life activities (sometimes referred to in the regulations as an "actual disability")." If a disability is not obvious to an employer, they can ask for medical documentation from a health care provider to confirm the need for an accommodation.

Individuals who solely are "regarded as" having a disability but do not have a disability, are not qualified to receive reasonable accommodations.

What Are "Essential Functions?"

In order to be qualified for a position, an applicant or employee must be able to perform essential job functions. Essential functions are job duties that are fundamental to the position, they are the reason the job exists. Some of the factors for determining essential functions of a job include:

1 Whether the position exists specifically to perform these essential functions.
2 The number of other employees who are available to perform the same job duties.
3 The expertise or skills required to perform the essential functions.

Obligations of Employers

What Types of Employers are Required to Provide Reasonable Accommodations?

Under the Americans with Disabilities Act, employers who have 15 or more employees are usually required to provide reasonable accommodations. Some state and local laws may require that employers with fewer employees provide reasonable accommodations.

Reasonable Accommodations Come in Many Forms

In order to determine what is reasonable, an employer must look at the request made by the applicant or employee with a disability. Whether or not an accommodation is reasonable will vary according to the position the employee holds, the way their disability affects their ability to do their job, and the environment that they work in.

What Types of Accommodations are Generally Considered Reasonable?

1   Change job tasks.
2   Provide reserved parking.
3   Improve accessibility in a work area.
4   Change the presentation of tests and training materials.
5   Provide or adjust a product, equipment, or software.
6   Allow a flexible work schedule.
7   Provide an aid or a service to increase access.
8   Reassign to a vacant position.

What Are Some Examples of Reasonable Accommodation?

Provide Alternative Formats: A supervisor gives feedback in writing, rather than verbally, for an employee who communicates better through written materials.

Accessible Parking: An employer changes its practice of only offering parking to upper management to allow an employee who is unable to walk long distances access to a reserved parking spot close to the building.

Service Animals: An employer reasonably changes their office's "no animals" policy, in order to welcome an employee's service animal.

Equipment Change: An employer purchases software that magnifies the computer screen to allow an employee with low vision to correctly enter and read information on the computer.

Reorganization of the Job: The employer provides a checklist to ensure task completion for an employee who has an intellectual disability.

Reassignment: Reassignment is the reasonable accommodation in some situations. An employer may reassign an employee to an open position if the employee can no longer perform the essential functions of their current job. **The employer does not have to create a new position, no other**

employees need be transferred or terminated in order to make a position vacant for the purpose of reassignment, and the individual with a disability should be qualified for the new position.

Reasonable Accommodation Process

According to the Equal Employment Opportunity Commission (EEOC) and Title I of the ADA, each request for a reasonable accommodation must be considered on a case-by-case basis. This section reviews the phases of the reasonable accommodation process. The first step in the reasonable accommodation process is disclosure of a disability, as employers are only required to accommodate disabilities of which they are aware. It is important to note that the process must be interactive, with participation by both the person with a disability and the employer, so that an effective solution may be agreed upon.

Get the Process Started

After an employee discloses a disability to their manager or to human resources, it is important to initiate whatever reasonable accommodation process that the employer has in place. Disclosure usually takes the form of: because of my disability(s),I am having trouble with X job duty or benefit or priviledge of employment. For an employee to disclose that they have a disability without also saying that it is impacting their work is usually not sufficient to begin the accommodation process. Disability disclosure should never be ignored.

Initiate an Interactive Dialog between the Employer and the Employee

The goal of this dialog is to understand what barrier the person is experiencing and why. It is also helpful to see if the person has any ideas about what might be useful for them. At this point, the employer can also provide an overview of the process, so the person who requested an accommodation understands what will happen next and who will have access to the information shared. All participants involved must agree to maintain confidentiality when discussing accommodations; reasonable accommodation information may only be shared on a need-to-know basis, will never go in a personnel file, and will not be shared with coworkers. Co-workers who may need to do something differently as a result of an accommodation may be told of the change required, but not the reasons why the change was made.

If Necessary, Obtain Preliminary Documentation

If the need for an accommodation is not obvious, the employee may be required to provide documentation of a disability from the appropriate health or rehabilitation professional.

The Accommodation Must be Effective

Both the employer and the employee are important participants in the process of finding an effective accommodation. The employee often knows what accommodation(s) will work best, because they know the barriers presented by their disability. The employer should participate, as they are familiar with the systems, policies, and practices in place within the organization. In the end, it is the employer who decides what accommodation is put into place, but it must be effective in resolving the functional limitation(s) presented by the disability.

Implement the Agreed Upon Reasonable Accommodation

Once the employer identifies an effective accommodation, make a plan to put it into effect on the job, including any necessary training for the employee. If an employer plans to deny an accommodation request, they should have a prepared reason for denying the request to give to the employee.

The Interactive Accommodation Process Should be Ongoing

The employer and the employee should continue communication to determine if the accommodations are working and make adjustments accordingly.

Document Dates, Actions taken, and Adjustments made to Assure Continued Success

All parties involved should document information about the reasonable accommodation process in order to maintain an accurate record and so that they can review the process and know what they have done to act on the accommodation.

Resources

ADA National Network

800-949-4232
www.adata.org

The Job Accommodation Network (JAN)

800-526-7234
www.askjan.org

Equal Employment Opportunity Commission (EEOC) ADA Information Line

800-669-4000 (Voice)
800-669-6820 (TTY)
www.eeoc.gov

For the most current and accessible version of this handout, please visit https://adainfo.us/accommodations

Appendix B: Assessment Scales

Contents:

260 ... Progress Tracker
261 ... Organization Time Management Planning (OTMP) measure
265 ... Durand Organizational Skills Questionnaire (DOSQ)
270 ... Time Management Scale-Revised (TMS-R)
273 ... Toronto Mindfulness Scale (Trait version)
275 ... Toronto Mindfulness Scale (State version)
277 ... Interpersonal Competence Questionnaire
281 ... Conflict Resolution Inventory
283 ... Parental Authority Questionnaire

Progress Tracker

Name: _____ Date: _____

Respond to the items based on how often they happened for you in the past week, using the following scale:

0 = Never/Not at all, 1 = Sometimes/Somewhat, 2 = Often/Much, 3 = Very often/Very Much

If there are "no problems" in an area because it is not applicable to your situation, leave it blank.

1	I have difficulty with attendance or being late at school or work	0	1	2	3
2	I have difficulty keeping appointments (doctor, professor, etc.)	0	1	2	3
3	I have trouble keeping track of when tests are scheduled or when assignments are due	0	1	2	3
4	I have difficulty getting to bed at a reasonable time.	0	1	2	3
5	I have problems getting ready to leave for the day	0	1	2	3
6	Others do important things for me (parents, friends, roommates, etc.)	0	1	2	3
7	I have problems getting work done efficiently (completing assignments, etc).	0	1	2	3
8	I have problems getting started on tasks at school and/or work	0	1	2	3
9	I have problems working to my potential (assignments are rushed or missing, etc.).	0	1	2	3
10	I use the internet, social media, video games, or TV excessively or inappropriately.	0	1	2	3
11	I have problems keeping up with chores (laundry, dishes, shopping, etc.)	0	1	2	3
12	I have problems managing money (paying bills on time, sticking to my budget, etc.).	0	1	2	3

Total of item responses: _____ **/ # items answered =** _____
IMPAIRMENT SCORE

Organization, Time Management, and Planning (OTMP) Self-Report Measure

Name: Date:

Do you have a system (e.g., calendar or planner) that you regularly use to schedule appointments or events?

                    Yes   No

If you answered "Yes" above, is your appointment scheduling system electronic or paper?

                    Electronic   Paper   Both

If you answered "Yes" above, please describe your appointment scheduling system:

Do you have a system (e.g., to-do list or task list) that you regularly use to manage or organize tasks you need to complete?

                    Yes   No

If you answered "Yes" to #3, is your to-do list system electronic or paper?

                    Electronic   Paper   Both

If you answered "Yes" to #3, is your to-do list system the same or different from your appointment system?

                    Same   Different

If you answered "Yes" to #4, please describe your to-do list system:

Please describe how you use technology to implement organization, time management, and planning skills into your life

How important is using technology in implementing these skills?

*Answer the following, using the stem "**During the last week, how often did**
you ..." for each item.*
Scale: *Never (0), Sometimes (1), Often (2), Very Often (3), Not applicable (NA)*

1   Add an appointment or event to your appointment scheduling system (e.g., class, doctor's appointment, concert or sporting event)

　　　　　　　　　　　　0　　　1　　　2　　　3　　　NA

2   Add a note to your appointment scheduling system (e.g., assignment or project due date, friend's birthday, reminder to pay bill, reminder to ask a particular question at a meeting or in class)

　　　　　　　　　　　　0　　　1　　　2　　　3　　　NA

3   Look at your appointment scheduling system to check your schedule.

　　　　　　　　　　　　0　　　1　　　2　　　3　　　NA

4   Look at your appointment scheduling system to check your availability for a particular day or time

　　　　　　　　　　　　0　　　1　　　2　　　3　　　NA

5   Add a task to your to-do list system (e.g., phone call, do laundry)

　　　　　　　　　　　　0　　　1　　　2　　　3　　　NA

6   Complete something from your to-do list system (e.g., finished assignment)

　　　　　　　　　　　　0　　　1　　　2　　　3　　　NA

7   Add an appointment to your appointment scheduling system to set aside time to complete something from your to-do list system (e.g., complete assignment after class and before going to the gym)

　　　　　　　　　　　　0　　　1　　　2　　　3　　　NA

8   Choose a task to complete from your to-do list system based on how urgent and/or important you thought the task to be

　　　　　　　　　　　　0　　　1　　　2　　　3　　　NA

9   Intentionally complete a higher priority (i.e., more urgent and/or important) task before a lower priority task (i.e., less urgent and/or important)

　　　　　　　　　　　　0　　　1　　　2　　　3　　　NA

10 Complete a lower priority task because you were having trouble with motivation and thought it was better to get something done

0   1   2   3   NA

11 Complete an enjoyable task when you knew you should have been doing something else (e.g., watched Netflix when you should have been doing your homework)

0   1   2   3   NA

12 Break down a large task (e.g., preparing for a final exam, writing a research paper) into more manageable tasks (e.g., scheduling 1-hour study sessions, creating deadlines to complete portions of paper)

0   1   2   3   NA

13 Check the time while completing an activity to make sure that you weren't going to be late for your next appointment or responsibility

0   1   2   3   NA

14 Hold yourself accountable by not letting yourself do something enjoyable until you finished a difficult task (e.g., didn't watch Netflix until you finished reading a chapter in my textbook)

0   1   2   3   NA

15 Organize your study or work area or materials (e.g., desk, backpack)

0   1   2   3   NA

16 Give yourself a reward after completing a portion of your academic tasks (e.g., went for a walk after finishing one section of your paper)

0   1   2   3   NA

17 Use waiting time or down time strategically to get small tasks done

0   1   2   3   NA

18 Immediately complete a brief task rather than adding it in your to-do list system

0   1   2   3   NA

19   Read your e-mails

0   1   2   3   NA

20   Sort and/or delete your e-mails

0   1   2   3   NA

21   Respond to your e-mails

0   1   2   3   NA

22   Complete a multi-step task (e.g., term paper, home improvement project) that was reflected in your to-do list items

0   1   2   3   NA

23   Complete tasks with deadlines that are on your to-do list on time or early

0   1   2   3   NA

24   Arrive at appointments (items in your calendar) on time

0   1   2   3   NA

25   Complete daily personal care tasks (e.g., brushing teeth, showering, laundry, dishes, cooking)

0   1   2   3   NA

26   Successfully find needed materials for tasks at home, school, or work (e.g., checkbook, class handouts, assignment instructions)

0   1   2   3   NA

27   Generally feel on top of the things that are going on and that you need to do in your life

0   1   2   3   NA

From: Canu, W. H., Knouse, L. E., Flory, K., & Hartung, C. M. (2023). *Thriving in College with ADHD: A Cognitive-Behavioral Skills Approach – Therapist Guide*

Durand Organizational Skills Questionnaire (DOSQ)

This questionnaire contains a series of 38 statements. In this questionnaire, the term 'work' is used to describe school, voluntary work, and employment. Answer the following statements according to the place where you spend most of your time and energy; whether it is going to school, doing voluntary work, or being employed. Describe yourself as you generally are now, not as you wish to be in the future. Describe yourself as honestly as you can.

For each statement please indicate by circling the appropriate number whether you:

Strongly disagree (1) with the statement - **Disagree** (2) with the statement - **Slightly disagree** (3) with the statement

OR

Slightly agree (4) with the statement – **Agree** (5) with the statement – **Strongly agree** (6) with the statement

There is no time limit to this questionnaire, but your first responses tend to be the most accurate.

1 I have a system to keep my books, notes, and other materials organized

       1 2 3 4 5 6

2 I feel that I have a tendency to forget important events (meetings, deadlines, etc.)

       1 2 3 4 5 6

3 I feel that I cannot work efficiently when my workspace is crowded with papers and junk

       1 2 3 4 5 6

4 It is often difficult for me to stay on track when I have to deal with a difficult long-term project

       1 2 3 4 5 6

5 I feel satisfied when my workplace is in order

       1 2 3 4 5 6

6 I rarely bother organizing e-mails and paperwork

       1 2 3 4 5 6

7 My colleagues would say that I am punctual

       1 2 3 4 5 6

8   Most of my work supplies are kept in the same place

1   2   3   4   5   6

9   I feel that many people often misunderstand what I am trying to say

1   2   3   4   5   6

10   I consider myself to be a punctual person

1   2   3   4   5   6

11   I keep track of where my documents are, even months after last working on them

1   2   3   4   5   6

12   It is often difficult for me to communicate my thoughts and ideas verbally to coworkers

1   2   3   4   5   6

13   I use various strategies to avoid being disorganized, such as keeping a detailed agenda

1   2   3   4   5   6

14   I rarely make a fully detailed schedule of the work I need to do on long term assignments with far away deadlines

1   2   3   4   5   6

15   I rarely leave tasks to the last minute

1   2   3   4   5   6

16   I generally have clear, personal, goals and objectives for myself at work

1   2   3   4   5   6

17   In general, my workspace is very messy

1   2   3   4   5   6

18   I use tools and systems (highlighters, charts, outlines, etc.) whenever I need to learn or gather new information

1   2   3   4   5   6

19 Whenever I decide to clean my workspace, it only stays clean for a few days or less

        1   2   3   4   5   6

20 I know exactly what I want to accomplish throughout my career

        1   2   3   4   5   6

21 I often misplace small objects

        1   2   3   4   5   6

The following questions pertain to your life outside work. Please respond to each statement with your personal life in mind, using the same scale as noted above.

22 I keep an organizer, such as a notebook or agenda, near me to write down important things I need to do

        1   2   3   4   5   6

23 I tend to lose important information, such as usernames, passwords, I.D. numbers, etc.

        1   2   3   4   5   6

24 I almost never set goals in my personal life

        1   2   3   4   5   6

25 In case of an emergency, I know exactly where I should look to get all my important documents

        1   2   3   4   5   6

26 When I need to sit down and work, I am able to motivate myself to do so

        1   2   3   4   5   6

27 I feel that people listening to me are often very confused

        1   2   3   4   5   6

28 My friends and family would consider me a punctual person

        1   2   3   4   5   6

29 I can easily visualize what I want to achieve in life

        1   2   3   4   5   6

30   I often change plans because I am overbooked due to underestimating the amount of time I need to complete a task

1	2	3	4	5	6

31   I am often misunderstood when I communicate with others

1	2	3	4	5	6

32   I often leave, or forget, some of my things at other people's places or in common areas

1	2	3	4	5	6

33   I regularly use an agenda to keep track of what to do, and when

1	2	3	4	5	6

34   Other people often have difficulties understanding what I mean

1	2	3	4	5	6

35   Whenever I start a chore, I often stop midway, for no particular reason

1	2	3	4	5	6

36   I often get confused when I interact with other people

1	2	3	4	5	6

37   It annoys me to see disorder around me

1	2	3	4	5	6

38   I find it difficult to stay on a schedule and get my chores done in a timely manner

1	2	3	4	5	6

Durand, G. (2020). *Measuring organizational skills in the general population: Development and preliminary validation of the DOSQ.* Preprints (www.preprints.org). https://www.preprints.org/manuscript/202008.0376/v1

Instructions to Clinicians for DOSQ Use

(Durand, 2020; personal communication, Guillaume Durand, May 20, 2022)

Items are rated from 1 (Strongly Disagree) to 6 (Strongly Agree)

Reverse code the following items:

2 + 4 + 6 + 9 + 12 + 14 + 17 + 19 + 21 + 23 + 24 + 27 + 30 + 31 + 32 + 34 + 35 + 36 + 38

Work organization: 8 + 11 + 25
Communication clarity: 9 + 12 + 27 + 31 + 34 + 36
Punctuality: 7 + 10 + 28
Goal-oriented: 16 + 20 + 24 + 29
Assiduity: 4 + 15 + 26 + 30 + 35 + 38
Workspace organization: 3 + 5 + 17 + 19 + 37
Strategies: 1 + 6 + 13 + 14 + 18 + 22 + 33
Attentiveness: 2 + 21 + 23 + 32
Total: sum of 8 scales

Durand, G. (2020). *Measuring organizational skills in the general population: Development and preliminary validation of the DOSQ.* Preprints (www.preprints.org). https://www.preprints.org/manuscript/202008.0376/v1

Personal communication, Guillaume Durand, May 20, 2022.

Time Management Scale – Revised (TMS-R)
Scale:

1 = never   2 = infrequently   3 = sometimes   4 = frequently   5 = always

Daily Planning subscale

1 Do you make a list of the things you have to do each day?

                          1   2   3   5   5

2 Do you plan your day before you start it?

                          1   2   3   4   5

3 Do you make a schedule of the activities you have to do on work days?

                          1   2   3   4   5

4 Do you write a set of goals for yourself each day?

                          1   2   3   4   5

5 Do you spend time each day planning?

                          1   2   3   4   5

6 Do you have a clear idea of what you want to accomplish during the next week?

                          1   2   3   4   5

7 Do you set and keep priorities?

                          1   2   3   4   5

Confidence in Long Term Planning subscale

8 Do you often find yourself doing things which interfere with your studying simply because you hate to say "No" to people?*

                          1   2   3   4   5

9 Do you believe that there is room for improvement in the way you manage your time?*

                          1   2   3   4   5

10 Do you make constructive use of your time?

1   2   3   4   5

11 Do you continue to carry out unprofitable routines or activities?*

1   2   3   4   5

12 Do you have a set of goals for the entire term?

1   2   3   4   5

13 Are you still working on a major assignment the night before it is due?*

1   2   3   4   5

14 Do you regularly review your lecture notes, even when a test is not imminent?

1   2   3   4   5

Notes for clinicians for TMS-R use

*: item is *reverse-scored*

College student norms M (SD; see Trueman & Hartley, 1995)

Men: Daily Planning 12.0 (3.9), Confidence in Long-term Planning 25.8 (5.8), Total 37.7 (7.8)

Women: Daily Planning 15.0 (4.1), Confidence in Long-term Planning 26.7 (4.5), Total 41.7 (7.1)

Toronto Mindfulness Scale (*Trait version*)

Instructions: We are interested in what you typically experience in your daily life. Below is a list of things that people sometimes experience. Please read each statement. Next to each statement are five choices: "not at all," "a little," "moderately," "quite a bit," and "very much." Please indicate the extent to which you agree with each statement. In other words, how well does the statement describe what you tend to experience in your daily life.	**Not at all**	**A little**	**Moder-ately**	**Quite a bit**	**Very much**
1 I experience myself as separate from my changing thoughts and feelings.	0	1	2	3	4
2 I am more concerned with being open to my experiences than controlling or changing them.	0	1	2	3	4
3 I am curious about what I might learn about myself by taking notice of how I react to certain thoughts, feelings or sensations.	0	1	2	3	4
4 I experience my thoughts more as events in my mind than as a necessarily accurate reflection of the way things 'really' are.	0	1	2	3	4
5 I am curious to see what my mind was up to from moment to moment.	0	1	2	3	4
6 I am curious about each of the thoughts and feelings that I was having.	0	1	2	3	4
7 I am receptive to observing unpleasant thoughts and feelings without interfering with them.	0	1	2	3	4
8 I am more invested in just watching my experiences as they arise, than in figuring out what they could mean.	0	1	2	3	4
9 I approach each experience by trying to accept it, no matter whether it was pleasant or unpleasant.	0	1	2	3	4

(Continued)

10	I remain curious about the nature of each experience as it arises.	0	1	2	3	4
11	I am aware of my thoughts and feelings without overidentifying with them.	0	1	2	3	4
12	I am curious about my reactions to things.	0	1	2	3	4
13	I am curious about what I might learn about myself by just taking notice of what my attention gets drawn to.	0	1	2	3	4

Scoring:

Key: All items were written in the positively keyed direction, so no reverse scoring of items is required.

Curiosity score: The following items are summed: 3, 5, 6, 10, 12, 13

Decentering score: The following items are summed: 1, 2, 4, 7, 8, 9, 11

Toronto Mindfulness Scale (*State version*)

Instructions: We are interested in what you just experienced. Below is a list of things that people sometimes experience. Please read each statement. Next to each statement are five choices: "not at all," "a little," "moderately," "quite a bit," and "very much." Please indicate the extent to which you agree with each statement. In other words, how well does the statement describe what you just experienced, just now?	**Not at all**	**A little**	**Moder-ately**	**Quite a bit**	**Very much**
1 I experienced myself as separate from my changing thoughts and feelings.	0	1	2	3	4
2 I was more concerned with being open to my experiences than controlling or changing them.	0	1	2	3	4
3 I was curious about what I might learn about myself by taking notice of how I react to certain thoughts, feelings or sensations.	0	1	2	3	4
4 I experienced my thoughts more as events in my mind than as a necessarily accurate reflection of the way things 'really' are.	0	1	2	3	4
5 I was curious to see what my mind was up to from moment to moment.	0	1	2	3	4
6 I was curious about each of the thoughts and feelings that I was having.	0	1	2	3	4
7 I was receptive to observing unpleasant thoughts and feelings without interfering with them.	0	1	2	3	4
8 I was more invested in just watching my experiences as they arise, than in figuring out what they could mean.	0	1	2	3	4
9 I approached each experience by trying to accept it, no matter whether it was pleasant or unpleasant.	0	1	2	3	4

(*Continued*)

10	I remained curious about the nature of each experience as it arose.	0	1	2	3	4
11	I was aware of my thoughts and feelings without overidentifying with them.	0	1	2	3	4
12	I was curious about my reactions to things.	0	1	2	3	4
13	I was curious about what I might learn about myself by just taking notice of what my attention gets drawn to.	0	1	2	3	4

Scoring:

Key: All items were written in the positively keyed direction, so no reverse scoring of items is required.

Curiosity score: The following items are summed: 3, 5, 6, 10, 12, 13

Decentering score: The following items are summed: 1, 2, 4, 7, 8, 9, 11

Interpersonal Competency Questionnaire

Instructions: Indicate your level of competence and comfort in handling each type of situation, by checking one box on the 5-point rating scale, where:

1 = I'm poor at this; I'd feel so uncomfortable and unable to handle this situation, I'd avoid it if possible;

2 = I'm only fair at this; I'd feel uncomfortable and would have lots of difficulty handling this situation;

3 = I'm OK at this; I'd feel somewhat uncomfortable and have some difficulty handling this situation;

4 = I'm good at this; I'd feel quite comfortable and able to handle this situation;

5 = I'm EXTREMELY good at this; I'd feel very comfortable and could hand this situation very well

		1 – Poor	2 – Fair	3 – OK	4 – Good	5 – Extremely Good
1	Asking or suggesting to someone new that you get together and do something (e.g., go out together).					
2	Telling a companion you don't like a certain way he or she has been treating you.					
3	Revealing something intimate about yourself while talking with someone you're just getting to know.					
4	Helping a close companion work through his or her thoughts and feelings about a major life decision (e.g., a career choice).					
5	Being able to admit that you might be wrong when a disagreement with a close companion begins to build into a serious fight.					
6	Finding and suggesting things to do with new people whom you find interesting and attractive.					

(Continued)

7	Saying "no" when a date/acquaintance asks you to do something you don't want to do.				
8	Confiding in a new friend/date and letting him or her see your softer, more sensitive side.				
9	Being able to patiently and sensitively listen to a companion "let off steam" about outside problems s/he is having.				
10	Being able to put begrudging (resentful) feeling aside when having a fight with a close companion.				
11	Carrying on conversations with someone new whom you think you might like to get to know.				
12	Turning down a request by a companion that is unreasonable.				
13	Telling a close companion things about yourself that you're ashamed of.				
14	Helping a close companion get to the heart of a problem s/he is experiencing.				
15	When having a conflict with a close companion, really listening to his or her complaints and not trying to "read" his/her mind.				
16	Being an interesting and enjoyable person to be with when first getting to know people.				
17	Standing up for your rights when a companion is neglecting you or being inconsiderate.				
18	Letting a new companion get to know the "real you."				
19	Helping a close companion cope with family or room-mate problems.				
20	Being able to take a companion's perspective in a fight and really understand his or her point of view.				
21	Introducing yourself to someone you might like to get to know (or date).				

(*Continued*)

22	Telling a date/acquaintance that he or she is doing something that embarrasses you.				
23	Letting down your protective "outer shell" and trusting a close companion.				
24	Being a good and sensitive listener for a companion who is upset.				
25	Refraining from saying things that might cause a disagreement to build into a big fight.				
26	Calling (on the phone) a new date/acquaintance to set up a time to get together and do something.				
27	Confronting your close companion when he or she has broken a promise.				
28	Telling a close companion about the things that secretly make you feel anxious or afraid.				
29	Being able to say and do things to support a close companion when s/he is feeling down.				
30	Being able to work through a specific problem with a companion without resorting to global accusations ("you always do that").				
31	Presenting good first impressions to people you might like to become friends with (or date).				
32	Telling a companion that he or she has done something to hurt your feelings.				
33	Telling a close companion how much you appreciate and care for him or her.				
34	Being able to show genuine empathetic concern even when a companion's problem is uninteresting to you.				
35	When angry with a companion, being able to accept and s/he has a valid point of view even if you don't agree with that view.				
36	Going to parties or gatherings where you don't know people well in order to start up new relationships.				
37	Telling a date/acquaintance that he or she has done something that made you angry.				

(Continued)

38	Knowing how to move a conversation with a date/ acquaintance beyond superficial talk to really get to know each other.					
39	When a close companion needs help and support, being able to give advice in ways that are well received.					
40	Not exploding at a close companion (even when it is justified) in order to avoid a damaging conflict.					

5 Subscales of ICQ:

Initiation: 1 + 6 + 11 + 16 + 21 + 26 + 31 + 36 = _____ / 8 = average score = _____
Negative Assertion: 2 + 7 + 12 + 17 + 22 + 27 + 32 + 37 = _____ / 8 = average score = _____
Disclosure: 3 + 8 + 13 + 18 + 23 + 28 + 33 + 38 = _____ / 8 = average score = _____
Emotional Support: 4 + 9 + 14 + 19 + 24 + 29 + 34 + 39= _____ / 8 = average score = _____
Conflict Management: 5 + 10 + 15 + 20 + 25 + 30 +35 + 40= _____ / 8 = average score = _____

Note: Average scores can be interpreted using the overall scale anchors (range 1 – 5), with higher scores indicating stronger skills. Some sex differences may be expected, as can differences depending on whether the person is mainly considering friends or their romantic partner(s). See Buhrmester et al. (1998) for further detail.

Conflict Resolution Styles Inventory

Instructions: Using the scale 1 = *Never* to 5 = *Always*, rate how frequently you use each of the following styles to deal with arguments or disagreements with your partner.

1 Launching personal attacks.

                1   2   3   4   5

2 Exploding and getting out of control.

                1   2   3   4   5

3 Getting carried away and saying things that aren't meant.

                1   2   3   4   5

4 Throwing insults and digs.

                1   2   3   4   5

5 Focusing on the problem at hand.

                1   2   3   4   5

6 Sitting down and discussing differences constructively.

                1   2   3   4   5

7 Finding alternatives that are acceptable to each of us.

                1   2   3   4   5

8 Negotiating and compromising.

                1   2   3   4   5

9 Remaining silent for long periods of time.

                1   2   3   4   5

10 Reaching a limit, "shutting down," and refusing to talk any further.

                1   2   3   4   5

11 Tuning the other person out.

                                    1   2   3   4   5

12 Withdrawing, acting distant and not interested.

                                    1   2   3   4   5

13 Not being willing to stick up for myself.

                                    1   2   3   4   5

14 Being too compliant.

                                    1   2   3   4   5

15 Not defending my position.

                                    1   2   3   4   5

16 Giving in with little attempt to present my side of the issue.

                                    1   2   3   4   5

Conflict engagement sum items 1–4:   _____

Positive problem solving sum items 5–8:   _____

Withdrawal sum items 9–12:   _____

Compliance sum items 13–16:   _____

Higher scores indicate greater use of that specific conflict resolution strategy.

Parental Authority Questionnaire

Parental Authority Questionnaire (PAQ)

Instructions: For each of the following statements, circle the number on the 5-point scale (**1 = *strongly disagree*, 5 = *strongly agree***) that best describes how the statement applies to you and your parent(s). Try to read and think about each statement as it applies to you and your parent(s) during your years of growing up at home. There are no right or wrong answers, so don't spend a lot of time on any one item. We are looking for your overall impression regarding each statement. Be sure not to omit any items. If your parents had significantly different approaches to parenting, we recommend completing this form separately for each one to get a better picture of your experience.

1 While I was growing up my parent(s) felt that in a well-run home the children should have their way in the family as often as the parents do.

1   2   3   4   5

2 Even if their children didn't agree with them, my parent(s) felt that it was for our own good if we were forced to conform to what they thought was right.

1   2   3   4   5

3 Whenever my parent(s) told me to do something as I was growing up, they expected me to do it immediately without asking any questions.

1   2   3   4   5

4 As I was growing up, once family policy had been established, my parent(s) discussed the reasoning behind the policy with the children in the family.

1   2   3   4   5

5 My parent(s) has always encouraged verbal give and take whenever I have felt that family rules and restrictions were unreasonable.

1   2   3   4   5

6   My parent(s) has always felt that what children need is to be free to make up their own minds and to do what they want to do, even if this does not agree with what their parents might want.

                    1   2   3   4   5

7   As I was growing up, my parent(s) did not allow me to question any decision they had made.

                    1   2   3   4   5

8   As I was growing up, my parent(s) directed the activities and decisions of the children in the family through reasoning and discipline.

                    1   2   3   4   5

9   My parent(s) has always felt that more force should be used by parents in order to get their children to behave the way they are supposed to.

                    1   2   3   4   5

10   As I was growing up, my parent(s) did not feel that I needed to obey rules and regulations of behavior simply because someone in authority had established them.

                    1   2   3   4   5

11   As I was growing up, I knew what my parent(s) expected of me in my family, but I also felt free to discuss those expectations with my parent(s) when I felt that they were unreasonable.

                    1   2   3   4   5

12   My parent(s) felt that wise parents should teach their children early who is boss in the family.

                    1   2   3   4   5

13   As I was growing up, my parent(s) seldom gave me expectations and guidelines for my behavior.

                    1   2   3   4   5

14　Most of the time as I was growing up my parent(s) did what the children in the family wanted when making family decisions.

$$1 \qquad 2 \qquad 3 \qquad 4 \qquad 5$$

15　As the children in my family were growing up, my parent(s) consistently gave us direction and guidance in rational and objective ways.

$$1 \qquad 2 \qquad 3 \qquad 4 \qquad 5$$

16　As I was growing up, my parent(s) would get very upset if I tried to disagree with them.

$$1 \qquad 2 \qquad 3 \qquad 4 \qquad 5$$

17　My parent(s) feels that most problems in society would be solved if parents would not restrict their children's activities, decisions, and desires as they are growing up.

$$1 \qquad 2 \qquad 3 \qquad 4 \qquad 5$$

18　As I was growing up, my parent(s) let me know what behavior they expected of me, and if I didn't meet those expectations, they punished me.

$$1 \qquad 2 \qquad 3 \qquad 4 \qquad 5$$

19　As I was growing up, my parent(s) allowed me to decide most things for myself without a lot of direction from them.

$$1 \qquad 2 \qquad 3 \qquad 4 \qquad 5$$

20　As I was growing up, my parent(s) took the children's opinions into consideration when making family decisions, but they would not decide for something simply because the children wanted it.

$$1 \qquad 2 \qquad 3 \qquad 4 \qquad 5$$

21　My parent(s) did not view themself as responsible for directing and guiding my behavior as I was growing up.

$$1 \qquad 2 \qquad 3 \qquad 4 \qquad 5$$

22   My parent(s) had clear standards of behavior for the children in our home as I was growing up, but they were willing to adjust those standards to the needs of each of the individual children in the family.

1   2   3   4   5

23   My parent(s) gave me direction for my behavior and activities as I was growing up and they expected me to follow their direction, but they were always willing to listen to my concerns and to discuss that direction with me.

1   2   3   4   5

24   As I was growing up my parent(s) allowed me to form my own point of view on family matters and she generally allowed me to decide for myself what I was going to do.

1   2   3   4   5

25   My parent(s) have always felt that most problems in society would be solved if we could get parents to strictly and forcibly deal with their children when they don't do what they are supposed to as they are growing up.

1   2   3   4   5

26   As I was growing up, my parent(s) often told me exactly what they wanted me to do and how she expected me to do it.

1   2   3   4   5

27   As I was growing up, my parent(s) gave me clear direction for my behaviors and activities, but they were also understanding when I disagreed with her.

1   2   3   4   5

28   As I was growing up, my parent(s) did not direct the behaviors, activities, and desires of the children in the family.

1   2   3   4   5

29 As I was growing up, I knew what my parent(s) expected of me in the family and they insisted that I conform to those expectations simply out of respect for their authority.

1   2   3   4   5

30 As I was growing up, if my parent(s) made a decision in the family that hurt me, they were willing to discuss that decision with me and admit if they made a mistake.

1   2   3   4   5

Parental prototype scores:

Permissive: 1 + 6 + 10 + 13 + 14 +17 + 19 + 21 + 24 + 28   = _____

Authoritarian: 2 + 3 + 7 + 9 + 12 + 16 + 18 + 25 + 26 + 29 = _____

Authoritative: 4 + 5 + 8 + 11 + 15 + 20 + 22 + 23 + 27 + 30 = _____

Index

Locators in **bold** refer to tables and those in *italics* to figures

academic accommodations 88–94
academic skills 70–86; communication
  with peers 85–86; communication
  with professors 81–85; distraction
  management 71–76; homework
  86, 89; memory strategies 76–79;
  note-taking strategies 79–81;
  practice planning 232, *233*
academic titles 82–85
accommodations, for persons with ADHD
  88–94, 227–228, 254–258
accountability, for completing tasks 52–59
activities of daily living *see* daily living
  activities
addressing academic tutors 82–85
adolescents, treatment responses
  22–23
'adulting' 208–209; *see also* daily living
  activities
alcohol 148–149, 242
Americans with Disabilities Act (ADA) **90**,
  228, 254
amphetamine 24, 26
app-based calendars 38–40
appointments, being organized about 214,
  220, 249, 253
assessment planning 2–3, 18–19
atomoxetine 24
attention-deficit/hyperactivity disorder
  (ADHD): assessment planning
  2–3, 18–19; causal and
  exacerbating factors **14**; cognitive-
  behavioral model *4*, 4–5, 96–99;
  in college students 1–2; educating
  clients 12–15; etiology **14**, 14–15;
  symptoms 3, 17; treatment of
  see treatment planning
attention, regulation of 16–18; *see also*
  self-regulation
attentional capacity 17
authoritarian parenting 197, 283–287
authoritative parenting 197, 283–287

behavioral routines 64–65

calendar and task list system: beginning
  and continuing to use 43–51;
  choice of 34–42
career exploration and planning 225–228;
  see also work
central nervous system (CNS) 24
classmates, communication with 85–86
client knowledge *see* educating clients
coaching metaphor 126–129
cognitive-behavioral model: of ADHD
  4–5, 96–99; effectiveness for
  students 23–24; noticing your
  patterns 114–122; thinking and
  responding differently 96–99
communication skills: for good
  relationships 180–182; listening
  skills 188–189; open
  communication 188; peers 85–86;
  professors 81–85; reciprocity 189
Conflict Resolution Inventory 281–282
conflict resolution skills 187–188
cultural factors 15

daily living activities 208–209; ADHD as
  related to 210–213; errands and

appointments 214, 220, 249, 253; financial management 214, 219, 248–249; grocery shopping and food preparation 213–214, 218–219, 247–248; living space and tidiness 213, 217–218, 247, 251; strategies for effectively managing 216–220, 247–253; travel and social plans 214, 220, 249–250, 253; work-related issues 215, 218, 221–228, 247

Daily Thought Record (DTR) 120–122, **130**, **137**, *235–236*

disabilities, accommodations for 88–94, 227–228, 254–258

distractions, and how to reduce 71–76

distributed practice 76, 77–78

driving safely 150, 166, 244

drug use 148–149, 156, 164–165, 242

Durand Organizational Skills Questionnaire (DOSQ) 265–268

eating *see* healthy eating

educating clients 10; ADHD, EF deficits, and other issues that impact concentration 11–19; psychosocial and medication treatments 21–28; task prioritization 55–56

email communication 83 85

emotional dysregulation 13, 96, 98

Emotional Support scales 185

emotions: cognitive model of ADHD 96–99; managing strong emotions and impulsive behavior 133–141; noticing your patterns 114–122; practicing new responses 123–131, *235–236*; procrastination 64; visualization of new responses 138–140

employment skills 222–228; *see also* work

executive function (EF): cognitive model of ADHD 96–97; deficits 15–16

exercise 147–148, 241

financial management 214, 219, 248–249, 253

the focus zone 71

food preparation 213–214, 218–219, 247–248, 252; *see also* nutrition

friendships 168–171

functional assessment 117–120, 124–125

gender differences in ADHD 14–15

grocery shopping 213–214, 218–219, 247–248, 252

group sessions 11

health *see* physical health; self-care

healthy eating *see* nutrition

homework: academic accommodations 94; academic skills 86, 89; calendar and task list systems 41–42, 44–46; daily living activities 215, 228; medication treatments 28; mindfulness 112; noticing your patterns 122; practicing new responses 124, 131, 140–141; procrastination 61, 66; relationships 193–194, 206–207; scheduling time for 49–51; self-care 150, 154, 157–158; task prioritization 53–54, 59

housework, being organized about 213, 217–218, 247, 251

hyperactivity 13

hyperactivity-impulsivity (HI) 185

impulsivity: educating clients 13; Emotional Support scales 185; managing strong emotions and impulsive behavior 133–141; practicing new responses 123–131

impulsivity inoculation 99

inattentive (IA) symptoms 185

Interpersonal Competence Questionnaire 277–280; *see also* relationships

job skills 222–228; *see also* work

laundry, being organized about 213, 217–218, 251

learning management system (LMS) 82

learning skills 67–69

lifestyle issues *see* exercise; nutrition; sleep

listening skills 188–189

meal planning 213–214

medication treatments 21–28

memory: note-taking strategies 79–81; strategies for remembering 76–79

mental well-being, link to physical health 142–143; *see also* self-care

methylphenidate 24

mindfulness 102–112, 273–276

mnemonics 76, 78–79
money, management of 214, 219,
        248–249, 253
monitoring *see* self-monitoring
Multimodal Treatment for ADHD (MTA)
        study 3

negative reinforcement 125
negative urgency 98
non-stimulant medications 24–25
note-taking strategies 79–81, 85
nutrition: goal setting 162–163, 237, 240;
        grocery shopping and food
        preparation 213–214, 218–219,
        247–248, 252; self-care
        146–147, 155

Oppositional Defiant Disorder and/or
        Conduct Disorder (ODD/CD) 197
organization, time management and
        planning (OTMP) skills: academic
        skills 71; background for the
        therapist 31–32; baseline skills
        32–33; becoming a professional
        learner 67–69; importance for
        people with ADHD 36–37;
        measures of 261–264; progress
        tracking **32**, 33, 260

Parental Authority Questionnaire
        283–287
parental relationships 169, 195–207
parenting styles 197
peers: changing behaviors 183–194;
        communication with 85–86;
        friendships 168–171
permissive parenting 197, 283–287
physical activity 147–148, 156,
        163–164, 241
physical health: exercise 147–148; health-
        related behaviors for goal setting
        153–158; link to mental well-being
        142–143; *see also* self-care
planning *see* organization, time
        management and planning
        (OTMP) skills; treatment planning
Pomodoro technique 75–76
positive urgency 98–99
prioritizing 52–59
procrastination and how to avoid it 60–66,
        71–76

professional learner skills 67–69
professors, communication with 81–85
progress tracking **32**, 33, 260
psychosocial treatments 21–28
psychotherapy 23–24

reciprocity 189
Red Flag Thoughts 125–126, 136
relationships: changing behaviors
        183–194; client discussions
        175–182; communication skills
        180–182; conflict resolution skills
        187–188; friendships 168–171;
        Interpersonal Competence
        Questionnaire 277–280; parental
        169, 195–207; romantic 169–170
rewards, and prioritising tasks 52–59
romantic relationships 169–170

Safren, S. A. 4, 126–127
scripts 64–65
self-care 142–145; health-related
        behaviors for goal setting
        153–158, 159–160; link between
        mental health and physical health
        142–143; nutrition 146–147, 155,
        162–163; physical activity
        147–148, 156, 163–164; sleep
        145–146, 155, 161–162; substance
        use 148–149, 156, 164–165;
        technology use 165–166
self-monitoring 106–107; Daily Thought
        Record (DTR) 120–122, **130**, **137**;
        form *234*; health-related behaviors
        158; noticing your patterns
        114–122; practicing new responses
        123–131, *235–236*; visualization of
        new responses 138–140
self-regulation 15–16; of attention 16–18;
        Red Flag Thoughts 125–126;
        thinking and responding
        differently 96–99
self-testing 76–77
sleep 145–146, 155, 161–162, 238–239
stimulant medications 24–26
student workbook 7–8
substance use 148–149, 156,
        164–165, 242

task list *see* calendar and task list system
task prioritization 52–59, 231

tasks of daily living *see* daily living activities
technology: ADHD as related to technology use 149–150, 165–166; app-based calendars 38–40; moderating use of 243
tidiness at home 213, 217–218, 247, 251
time management *see* organization, time management and planning (OTMP) skills; procrastination and how to avoid it
Time Management Scale-Revised (TMS-R) 270–272
time tracking 49
Toronto Mindfulness Scale 106, 273–276
treatment duration 6–7
treatment planning 2–3; cognitive-behavioral model 4–5; effectiveness for students 23–24; how is ADHD treated? 22–23; modular approach 5–7; psychosocial and medication treatments 21–28
tutors, communication with 81–85

visualization of new responses 138–139

well-being *see* self-care
work: accommodations for 227–228, 254–258; being organized about 215, 218, 250, 251–252; career exploration and planning 225–228; succeeding at 221–228

'the zone' 71